Models of Mental Disorders

A New Comparative Psychiatry

Models of Mental Disorders

A New Comparative Psychiatry

William T. McKinney, M.D.

University of Wisconsin Medical School
Madison, Wisconsin

PLENUM MEDICAL BOOK COMPANY
NEW YORK AND LONDON

Library of Congress Cataloging in Publication Data

McKinney, William T.
  Models of mental disorders.

  Includes bibliographies and index.
  1. Mental Illness—Animal models. 2. Animal psychopathology. 3. Psychiatry,
Comparative. I. Title. [DNLM: 1. Disease Models, Animal. 2. Mental Disorders. 3.
Psychopathology. WM 100 M4784]
RC455.4.A54M35   1988   616.89′00724   88-2335
ISBN-13: 978-1-4684-5432-1   e-ISBN-13: 978-1-4684-5430-7
DOI: 10.1007/978-1-4684-5430-7

© 1988 Plenum Publishing Corporation
Softcover reprint of the hardcover 1st edition 1988
233 Spring Street, New York, N.Y. 10013

Plenum Medical Book Company is an imprint of Plenum Publishing Corporation

Preface

My ideas for this book have been evolving over the last several years as I have been working in the animal modeling area and have seen it change rather dramatically. There have been tremendous advances, both in methodology and in conceptualization, yet the literature is scattered in journals encompassing many disciplines. In particular, there have been only very limited attempts to write about the philosophical, conceptual, and controversial issues in this field; to pull together diverse findings; and to provide some general perspective on its future.

As will probably be apparent, I am a clinical psychiatrist who also has a fundamental interest in animal behavior, especially primate social behavior. I entered the field from a clinical research standpoint to develop some animal models of depression after being stimulated to do so by Dr. William Bunney, then at the National Institute of Mental Health and now at the University of California–Irvine. The field has grown rapidly since then and there is considerable research activity. Indeed, the research activity has grown more rapidly than our conceptualization of what animal models are and are not.

Animal preparations are now available for studying specific aspects of certain types of psychopathology. Thoughtful workers in the animal modeling field no longer talk about comprehensive models but rather about more limited experimental preparations in animals for studying certain specific aspects of human psychopathology.

Despite the amount of research activity in this area, there is no integrated and easily available reference source for students and workers. This particular book is intended to be a discussion of some general philosophical issues concerning the development, evaluation, and uses of animal models in psychiatry, plus an overview of four selected areas of research in the animal modeling field. It would be impossible to be comprehensive and still have a book of manageable size. Rather, the attempt has been to give the reader some general idea of ongoing research in the area. I have tried to be scientifically accurate but not so technical that the worker or student from outside the field becomes lost. The syndromes selected—depression, schizophrenia, anxiety, and alcoholism—are used to illustrate some of the conceptual points made in the first few chapters. They are all areas of active research investigation, but of course others could have been included. One is the area of organic mental disorders. However, the techniques being used are fundamentally different from those being used to study the four syndromes discussed and seemed more appropriate as the subject of a separate monograph. Another important group of psychiatric disorders are those involving substance abuse. However, the discussion of animal models of substance abuse would occupy the full length of this book and more, since multiple drugs are involved and the techniques for studying the different drugs vary. The literature is enormous and, in my opinion, also deserves to be treated in a separate book.

The final section of the book is a synthesis of the key conceptual and controversial issues in the field of animal modeling. This chapter is timely because there is great tension between molecularly oriented neuroscientists and their conceptualization and expectations of animal models, and researchers whose major interest is in the study of ongoing social behavior. Particularly in this era of high-technology neuroscience, it is important to remember that behavior occurs in a developmental and social context and that, if one wants to understand the neurobiological underpinnings of behavior, existing techniques must be appropriately adapted and new ones developed to permit the combined study of behavior and neurobiology.

The author of any book of this scope must be indebted to many people for making it possible. As mentioned before, Dr. William Bunney stimulated my interest in this field in 1967. Dr. David Hamburg has been a continuing source of stimulation and support for my activities in this area. When I went to the University of Wisconsin in 1969, I had the opportunity to work closely with Dr. Harry Harlow, who personally made it possible for me to begin my work at the Wisconsin Primate Laboratory. Dr. Arthur Prange and Dr. Morris Lipton were my first two mentors in psychiatric research, and without them I would never have entered the field in the first place. I have been fortunate to have had very capable, high quality members in my research group over the years; with the unpredictability and uncontrollability of research funding in this controversial area, they deserve special commendation for their risk-taking.

This book was written while I was a Fellow at the Center for Advanced Studies in Behavioral Sciences at Stanford, California, in 1983–1984. I acknowledge with great thanks those at the University of Wisconsin–Madison and at the Center who made this important year possible. In particular I am grateful for financial support provided by the John D. and Catherine T. MacArthur Foundation and to Mardi Horowitz who read and commented on portions of the manuscript.

This book could not have been written without the cooperation and loving support of my family—Carolyn, Scott, and Julia—to whom this book is dedicated. They were uprooted from friends and home in Madison to come to a new place for a year so that I could have the time to think and to write about an exciting new area of research.

William T. McKinney

Madison, Wisconsin

Contents

III. *Perspectives on the Animal Modeling Field*

Introduction

This book is about animal models of psychiatric illnesses. It is oriented primarily toward clinicians, to provide an overview of a new and rapidly developing area of psychiatry, but with sufficient technical accuracy so that researchers in the area will also find it useful. The latter group can follow developments in this area by tracking relevant journals. However, the problem for clinicians who are not intimately involved with this research area is that the literature is widely scattered in journals that span experimental and developmental psychology, ethology, animal behavior, clinical psychiatry, primatology, psychopharmacology, and the neurosciences, to mention only a few examples.

There is no easily available reference source that combines an explanation of the basic conceptualizations behind animal modeling for psychiatric illnesses along with a discussion of illustrative work on several of the major forms of psychopathology. This is the major purpose of this book, namely, to provide for clinicians in several mental health areas, a basic understanding of the philosophy of animal models and to highlight trends with regard to four syndromes—affective disorders, anxiety disorders, the schizophrenias, and alcoholism.

Clinicians not active in this research area tend to make one of two mistakes concerning animal modeling research. They either over-embrace it, and are too quick to jump to clinical conclusions from a given set of animal behavior experiments, or they regard animal modeling research with disdain, viewing it as essentially irrelevant. Perhaps a third problem should be mentioned, namely, ignorance of an increasingly large body of work in the area. The above errors are understandable given the lack of an available reference source to aid in the basic understanding and evaluation of proposed approaches to modeling human psychopathology.

This book takes the position that in order to understand and evaluate a rapidly expanding literature in several areas of animal modeling research, there must first be a fundamental understanding of the basis and justification for having models. This must be coupled with a realization of the limitations of animal models in relation to psychiatric syndromes. The articulation and understanding of this fundamental philosophy is necessary to prevent both an uninformed rejection of animal modeling research or, on the other hand, an overacceptance of its clinical relevance. Therefore, in Part I this book has a heavy emphasis on a historical perspective for animal models and on the philosophical basis for animal model development. The key points that are developed in this part are the following:

1. The early history of the field was characterized by narrative descriptions of animal behavior with little attention to quantitative assessment. Clinical labels were used loosely, and methods to induce altered behavior in animals bore little resemblance to those thought to produce human psychopathology. The field of experimental psychopathology research and clinical psychiatry developed far apart despite the attempts of some creative workers to bridge the gap.

2. We now recognize that there is no such thing as a comprehensive animal model for any psychiatric syndrome. Basically, animal models should be viewed as experimental preparations developed in one species for the purpose of studying phenomena occurring in another species. The concern is with developing experimental paradigms to study selected aspects of human psychopathology, not to develop a "schizophrenic" or "alcoholic" animal. However, animals are now being creatively used to study selected issues about schizophrenia and alcoholism that cannot be studied in any other way.

3. There are at least four different kinds of animal models: (a) those designed to simulate specific signs or symptoms of the human disorder, (b) those designed to test specific etiological theories, (c) those designed to study underlying mechanisms, and (d) those designed to permit preclinical drug evaluation. Each of these is discussed in general and then in the context of each of the illustrative syndromes chosen in Part II.

4. In Part I there is also considerable discussion about the rationale for developing animal models in the first place, along with

guidelines for evaluating them. A related issue which is addressed is how to properly reason across species and thus be able to evaluate the signifiance of published data.

Part II of the book discusses four syndromes—affective disorders, anxiety disorders, schizophrenic disorders, and alcoholism. In the case of each syndrome, an overview of animal modeling research is provided. By and large, the details of the experimentation are not provided, and the original data are not presented. This is not the intent of this book. Rather, the goal is to provide, primarily for clinicians, an overview of approaches being used in each of the four areas that will illustrate the fundamental points made in Part I. Countless numbers of journal articles contain the original data, and this book attempts to do something else, namely, to provide a perspective on the field and some illustrative examples. Therefore, the reader should not necessarily expect Part II to be a comprehensive review. Even if it were at the time of writing, it would likely be dated by publication. Having said the above, an attempt is made to provide a representative cross section of research, not just one particular approach, in each of the syndromes chosen. Therefore, while not entirely comprehensive, it is hoped that this section is not parochial.

Why were these specific syndromes chosen? First, they each represent extremely important areas of clinical concern and activity. Second, there is a body of animal modeling research in each of the areas that could be used to illustrate the conceptual points made in the first part of the book in a manner that will be understandable. A few other syndromes could have been added, but the desire was to keep the length of this book reasonably short so that it would be more likely to be read.

Part III discusses what I think are some of the future tasks in the animal modeling research area. This is likely to be the most controversial part of the book but is being included because of its importance. Despite tremendous advances in the animal modeling research area and its great clinical relevance, its very future is in considerable jeopardy. The dangers relate not so much to the necessary scientific tasks, which are discussed in this section, but to some administrative and political issues, which are also dealt with. These range from attempts by some to shut down biomedical animal research altogether, to some significant political, organizational, and administrative issues within granting agencies. Some readers may find these issues too specific if they are not personally in the research area, although I am frequently impressed by the interest and capabilities of a broad range of clinical audiences to appreciate these problems and to be helpful in developing solutions. To my knowledge, the content of Part III, regarding future tasks, has never been organized in this manner. As with any document that attempts to outline future tasks, the danger is that they will have been successfully handled by the time the publication comes out. In this case, it is doubtful, but the prospect is a pleasant one to ponder.

I

Fundamental Basis and Justification for a New Comparative Psychiatry

1

Historical Perspective

Introduction

It is important early in the course of this book, which attempts to provide a conceptual framework for a new area of psychiatry, for the reader to gain a historical perspective on some early research relevant to later developments. If this is not done there is a danger that history will repeat itself. As will become apparent, this would not be all bad since there were some extremely important early contributions which laid the foundation for much of the current research activity in this area. However, there were also some major problems, including the fact that the early origins of what might be called "comparative psychiatry" actually began outside of clinical psychiatry and proceeded along a different pathway. The techniques and terminology were foreign to most clinicians, and there was a tendency either to ignore the emerging body of animal behavior research relevant to psychiatry or to overembrace it with a premature application of clinical labels to behaviors shown by animals in laboratory settings. Examples of these problems are given in this historical overview.

The detailed reading of the early history of this field can be quite tedious, and there is always the risk that by putting this chapter first I will lose some nonhistorically oriented readers. For this reason this chapter is kept short and written in such a way as to highlight trends rather than the details of experimental protocols. There is an attempt to explain what may be unfamiliar terms and to relate them to more current clinical terminology.

Readers may be surprised to find in this chapter some theoretical conceptualizations about human psychopathology, based in part on work with animals, that have been recently rediscovered as part of the "new neurobiology." Such is the danger of ignoring history! Rather than itemize these now I leave it to the readers to make their own list as this chapter is read.

At the end of this chapter, as well as all the chapters that follow, a summary of key points is provided.

History

Though Pavlov is often said to be the originator of research relevant to animal modeling of human psychopathology, Pavlov himself gives credit to E. L. Thorndike, who he says preceded him in this area by 3 years. He paraphrases Thorndike to the effect that it is more important to be acquainted with exact outward behavior of humans than with guesses about their internal states with all their combinations and changes (Pavlov, 1928). Thorndike went from this position to laboratory experiments on animals. However, the first extensive work in experimental psychopathology with animals was done in Russia in Pavlov's laboratory. As is often the case in the history of science, the experimental study of psychopathology was not the original aim of the research. Rather, Pavlov made serendipitous, or almost accidental, observations. For example, in Pavlov's laboratory, Shenger-Krestovnikova (1921) was conducting the now classic circle–ellipse experiment. In this experiment a dog was taught to discriminate a circle from an ellipse in order to get food. Gradually the circle and the ellipse came to look more and more like each other until a ratio of 9 : 8 was reached. At this point the dog's discrimination became poor and, after three weeks, broke down. The dog went from being quiet to being highly upset. It would no longer stay in it's experimental apparatus and violently resisted going into the test room. Even easy discriminations, which the dog previously solved readily, were disrupted. Right or wrong, Pavlov called this kind of behavior "experimental neurosis" and began to draw parallels between this state in his dogs and the various neuroses of humans (Pavlov, 1928, 1941).

Pavlov's definition of experimental neurosis merits some discussion. By neurosis he meant chronic deviation from normal in "higher nervous activity." In his framework, higher nervous activity consisted of conditioned positive and negative reflexes. By a positive reflex he meant a conditioned response to a stimulus predicting food, and by a negative reflex he meant a conditioned response to a stimulus predicting no food. Excitation in the cerebral cortex was inferred from positive reflexes, and inhibition, from negative reflexes. He felt that in neuroses there was a weakening of the excitatory and inhibitory processes and chaotic nervous activity. This might be thought of as a relatively primitive explanation by present day standards given the increased knowledge base in the neurosciences. However, when we examine current neurobiological research in the area of the neuroses we cannot help but be impressed by Pavlov's genius in anticipating the future. Pavlov also foresaw the role of temperament, traits, or personality in determining responses to stress. In this context he spoke of four types of dogs. Two types were "extreme" and two were "balanced." The extremes were either excitable (choleric) or inhibitory (melancholic). The balanced ones were either calm (phlegmatic) or lively (sanguine). He felt that the two extreme groups were the ones most susceptible to breakdown under stress.

He postulated that many factors interacted to produce altered behavior in the dogs. These factors included genetic and developmental factors, the nature of current stressors, and neurobiological status. We are slowly rediscovering some of these factors and how they interact to produce alterations in human, and animal, behavior. Pavlov also began the study of pharmacological agents in his dogs and helped develop this avenue of research, which has proved to be an important one in experimental psychopathology.

Of course, we now understand neurosis to be a heterogenous term which encompasses many different entities. It is unlikely that any unitary explanation, such as that developed by Pavlov, could fully explain all forms of neuroses. Nevertheless, he was a pioneer in highlighting certain principles. One of the most interesting aspects of Pavov is his attention to the interaction between personality "types" (probably a combination of genetic and developmental influences) and the management of ongoing stress. The current stress used in his, and some other earlier workers' paradigms, involved increasingly difficult discriminations in a conditioning paradigm. Today, these stressors include such things as uncontrollability, separations, treatment with pharmacological agents, and neurotoxic lesioning.

Based on his animal work, Pavlov developed a theory of human schizophrenia which is difficult for many to understand. However, his work with animals and his theoretical formulations have spawned much research on schizophrenia in Russia. These theoretical models of human psychopathology were derived from animal studies. Certain human observations were made based on these theoretical formulations, and clinical research with humans was subsequently undertaken. Whether or not the theoretical models were correct is a matter of some debate, but they did have considerable heuristic value. The key point to be made in this context is that animal studies can lead to the development of new theories regarding human psychopathology in addition to making it possible to evaluate certain existing theories.

It has been said that Pavlov's work represented the first move away from the correlational method of behavioral analysis to the experimental study of psychopathology.

> The significance of this change in direction may best be comprehended in relation to its two most important implications. First, the completely correlational method of behavioral analysis which was the empirical foundation of all earlier systematic efforts to understand psychological abnormality, including everything from Hippocrates' humors and Gall's prominences to the ingenious psychoanalytic theorizing of Freud, could now be supplemented if not altogether supplanted by a direct experimental approach which was much less fraught with the dual dangers of loose conjecture and empirical untestability. Second, and historically of possibly greater significance, the continuity of animal morphology, physiology, and behavior, already beginning to assume a position on center stage in man's philosophical thinking, received a new extensive thrust from the early Pavlovian findings since for the first time even such "uniquely human" phenomena as emotional breakdowns were seen to occur in subhuman animals. (Kimmel, 1971, p. 4)

Another early worker in the field of experimental psychopathology was W. Horseley Gantt (1944, 1971), who first met Pavlov during the Russian famine of 1922 when he was in the Soviet Union as a member of a medical relief team. Like Pavlov, he became interested in experimental neurosis as a result of a laboratory accident. About 15 dogs escaped from their cages in his laboratory and roamed all over the building barking and fighting. They subsequently showed disturbances of their conditioned reflexes and of other behaviors. One of these was the dog named Nick, whose case has been well described in the literature.

On the basis of his research with dogs, Gantt formulated two principles of psychopathological development, schizokinesis and autokinesis (Gantt, 1962). It is interesting that these terms are no longer used very much, at least not in the sense they were first used, but the concepts to which they refer have become increasingly important in our current understanding of psychopathology. *Schizokinesis* was originally defined by Gantt as being the discrepancy between emotional (visceral) components of the conditioned response and the external skeletal components, for example, the situation where there is no skeletal response but a continued heart rate increase to a stimulus that no longer elicits danger. *Autokinesis* was defined by Gantt as being the progressive, internal development of response in the absence of further external stimulation. Psychiatric clinicians will recognize both of these principles as fundamental ones in many forms of psychopathology. Gantt's contribution comes from the development of these concepts based on his work with animals, although he did not link them up very precisely with specific forms of psychopathology. The importance of animal work in this regard, that is, helping to develop and elucidate basic principles of psychopathology, is a theme developed many times in the course of this book. This contribution is more fundamental and important than whether a given set of behaviors in a given animal species does or does not accurately represent a specific human clinical syndrome in some global sense.

Liddell reported the first observation of experimental neurosis using sheep as subjects. Liddell and Bayne (1927) reported "experimental neurasthenia" in a sheep subjected to an unsignaled doubling of the number of conditioning trials per day. The animal became very excited and agitated. Liddell and his research group continued to perform experimental neurosis research on sheep, goats, and pigs using conditioning paradigms (Anderson and Parmenter, 1941; Liddell, 1947; Liddell, Anderson, Kotyuka, and Hartman, 1935). They developed the concept that experimental disorders in animals represented primitive, relatively undifferentiated behavioral states rather than one specific syndrome.

Another historical figure in the animal modeling field is Jules Masserman, who brought an extensive background in psychiatry and in psychoanalysis to experimental neurosis research. Working initially with cats, and then later with monkeys, he tried to demonstrate that phenomena similar to that described by Pavlov could be induced but by using different methods. (Masserman, 1943, 1971; Masserman, Arieff, Pechtel, and Klehr, 1950). He used laboratory conflict between motivations as his inducing technique. Specifically, animals were taught to associate a signal with the delivery of food into a food box. Then they were subjected to blasts of air or grid shocks when they responded to the signal. Masserman labeled the resultant behaviors "phobias." These behaviors included changes in spontaneous activity, crouching, hiding, trying to escape from the apparatus, and pulse and respiratory patterns indicative of fear. Sometimes the animals would show what could be called *counterphobic behaviors,* or what Masserman labeled stereotyped behaviors. They would also show "regressive" behaviors such as preening and playing. He also tried to develop methods to alleviate the abnormal behaviors produced.

Thus far in the history of the field of experimental neurosis we are dealing mostly with narrative descriptions by the investigator of the animals' behavior. Quantitative ratings of their behavior were, by and large, not being done. However, the development and utilization of highly sophisticated and quantifiable measurements of social behavior has evolved from these descriptions. As a result of these early narrative descriptions which, by the way, were often very literary and interesting, a variety of clinical terms, rather than descriptive ones, were developed to describe the animals' behavior. It is perhaps this overly liberal use of clinical terms, combined with the use of induction techniques which were unfamiliar to most clinicians, that led the field of experimental psychopathology to develop far apart from clinical psychiatry.

In any event, Masserman's work attracted considerable attention and led to the development of his four biodynamic principles, postulated to guide behavior (Masserman, 1961). These are the following: (a) the actions of all organisms are directed toward satisfying physiological needs; (b) organisms conceive of and interact with their milieu not in terms of an absolute reality but according to their genetic capacity, rates of maturation, and unique experience; (c) behavior is adaptive; (d) the development of neurotigenesis: when physical inadequacies, environmental stresses, or motivational conflicts exceed adaptive capacities, internal tensions mount (anxiety), neurophysiological (psychosomatic) dysfunctions occur, and the organism develops overgeneralized patterns of avoidance (phobias), stereotyped behavior (obsessions and compulsions), aberrant conspecific and extraspecific transactions (social deviations) and regressive, hyperactive, or hostile or bizarrely "dereistic" (hallucinations, delusions) responses analogous to those in human neuroses and psychoses. This conceptualization was later revised to explain neurosis-generating conflict conditions as part of broader principles of unpredictability and uncontrollability. This later modification is interesting in view of recent research in the learned helplessness area which also points to the importance of uncontrollability and the fact that such a state has many neurobiological as well as behavioral effects.

Again, it was not so much that Masserman simulated a specific human condition in animals; indeed, the inducing condition involving motivational conflict would at best be considered controversial as a generalized etiological factor for neuroses. There is even controversy in the literature about whether the effects seen were due to motivational conflict or to some artifacts of the experimental situation such as confinement. It is unlikely that this latter interpretation sufficiently accounts for all of his findings. However, the claims for symptom similarity between cat and human neurosis are not persuasive alone, and clinical terms are sometimes used so loosely that they become meaningless. Nevertheless, the biodynamic principles Masserman formulated, based in part on his animal work, have importance in our basic understanding of psychopathology.

Masserman later studied several primate species using inducing techniques involving sequential–temporal uncertainty and unpredictability. It is this work, illustrated by the following quote, which led to the revision of his fourth principle:

> . . . unpredictability may give existence its zest but also imbues it with an anxiety that can best be ameliorated by rendering life, friends, and future more nearly certain. (Masserman, 1971, p. 32)

The greatest contribution of Masserman's work lay not in its simulation of any particular behavioral state but in its demonstration that certain psychoanalytic principles can be made operational and tested experimentally. This was no small contribution in its time nor is it even today.

There have been other scattered reports of animal "neurosis." For example, Hebb's description of spontaneous neurosis in chimpanzees was important in terms of its relation to clinical and experimental phenomena. He described what he termed a "phobia" in one case in which a chimp suddenly became afraid of large chunks of food. The other case involved a naturally occurring depression (Hebb, 1947). Babkin (1938) reported that bromides could reset the balance between excitatory and inhibitory processes thought by Pavlov and Gantt to be important in experimental neuroses. Stainbrook (1947) called attention to the value of experimentally producing acute behavioral disorders in animals as a method of psychosomatic research and discussed some of the previous work done in several species. Cook (1939) and Dworkin *et al.* (1942) also published reports in this area.

It is difficult to know what conclusions to draw about this early history of the field of experimental psychopathology research. Many who have reviewed it have not seen it as an auspicious beginning. Yet a more careful look at the work of some of the early pioneers yields more than at first meets the eye. While they may have been unsuccessful in modeling specific syndromes, certain fundamental principles of importance that we are rediscovering today have come from this work. These have been mentioned throughout this chapter but, in summary, are as follows:

1. Early researchers demonstrated that psychopathology could be studied experimentally in animals in addition to the strictly correlational studies done previously in humans.
2. They demonstrated the importance of careful observations and of serendipity. While it is true that these early workers did not use the more sophisticated and quantifiable behavioral scoring

techniques now available, they were astute observers and literary describers.

3. An interactive model of psychopathology was strongly suggested by all of the previously discussed work. The role of the temperament of the animals, along with a number of other variables, was shown early to be an important factor in influencing responses to current stresses. This phenomenon is well illustrated by Pavlov's work, which found large individual variability in the response to conditioning paradigms. The sources of such variability continue to be an important area of investigation today, and animal studies continue to add greatly to our knowledge regarding these sources of variance.

4. The principle of a persistent internal response, even after the inducing stimulus is no longer present, is a major contribution in our understanding of a number of forms of psychopathology.

5. The importance of unpredictability and uncontrollability was recognized by these early workers although systematic investigations of this phenomenon are more recent.

6. As summarized by Kimmel (1971), the experimental paradigms exemplified another basic principle, namely, that adaptive behavioral processes provide the foundation on which maladaptive behavior patterns are built, given altered environmental demands. Adaptive mechanisms, of animals and humans, are fragile and share a tenuous relationship with the environment. Internal changes in the organism (e.g., with drugs or other altered neurochemistry) and/or changes in the external environment (e.g., separation or uncontrollability) can lead to serious behavioral changes. The study of these interactions is becoming a cornerstone of animal modeling research.

It is interesting that these workers focused largely on an ill-defined clinical category termed "experimental neuroses" (although Pavlov also talked about his work in relation to schizophrenia). This term was used imprecisely and the behaviors described were in large part unfamiliar to clinicians who were treating people with one or another of the disorders subsumed under this heading. On the other hand, clinical diagnostic criteria were not very precise at that time. Therefore, it was impossible to relate the behaviors shown by the animals to specific syndromes. This failure, I think, led to severe communication difficulties between animal behavior researchers and clinicians. It is illustrated by Kubie's criticism when he stated, "Thus the imitation in animals of the emotional states which attend neuroses in man is not the experimental production of the essence of neuroses itself" (Kubie, 1939).

Kubie's contention was that behavior was only the "sign language" of an underlying symbolic disorder which was the real core of psychopathology. He felt that animals do not have symbolic capacities, and, therefore, it is not possible to produce a true neurotic or psychotic state in nonhumans. This position is predicated on an assumption about human psychopathology that few would now agree with, namely, that behavior is important only as an indicator of the more important "real" disorder. Modern clinical diagnostic methods have moved well beyond this assumption and use a combination of phenomenological descriptions and history to make diagnoses. Also, the assumption that higher-order primates do not have symbolic capacities is a concept that most would reject today.

More recent animal modeling research has focused on the affective disorders, schizophrenia, and alcoholism more so than the neuroses, although some very interesting work, possibly relevant to our understanding of anxiety disorders, is now available. Each of these topics is covered in separate chapters of this book and additional relevant history discussed in this context rather than in the present chapter.

Summary of Key Points

- *Pavlov and Thorndike were early pioneers in research relevant to animal modeling of human psychopathology. Their work highlighted the importance of careful behavioral observations rather than speculations about the nature of internal states.*

- *Pavlov's work represented the first move away from the correlational method of behavioral analysis to the experimental study of psychopathology. He was one of the first to postulate a truly interactive model of psychopathology involving genetic and developmental factors in addition to current stressors and neurobiology. Such a model was based in large part on his work with animals in a laboratory setting.*

- *Research utilizing animals has been critical in developing and elucidating basic principles of psychopathology. This contribution has been a fundamental and important one, and it supercedes debates about whether or not a given set of behaviors in animals does or does not accurately represent a specific human clinical syndrome in some global sense.*

- *Various animals were used in the early history of the comparative psycho-pathology field, for example, dogs, sheep, primates, cats, goats, etc. There are advantages and limitations to each kind of animal, and these need to be carefully considered in designing studies. The choice of the animal should relate to the question being investigated rather than to other factors.*

- *In the early phases of the development of this field the literature was characterized by narrative, literary descriptions. Clinical terms were used far too loosely to describe the animals' behavior. Quantitative ratings of behavior evolved from these early descriptions and have gradually come to prevail in most research settings. One might add that the literary aspects are no longer well accepted.*

- *From a historical standpoint the preoccupation has been with "experimental neurosis" research in animals. What was meant by this terminology was not always clear and certainly seemed foreign to most clinicians. The case examples in Section II of this book will use syndromes which should be more clinically familiar—affective disorders, anxiety disorders, schizophrenia, and alcoholism. However, before discussing animal work relevant to each of these syndromes, it is necessary to have a conceptual basis for understanding the work. This is done in Chapter 2.*

References

Anderson, D. D., and Parmenter, R. (1941) A Long Term Study of the Experimental Neurosis in the Sheep and Dog. *Psychosomatic Medicine* 2–4:1–150.

Babkin, B. P. (1938) Experimental Neurosis in Animals and Their Treatment With Bromides. *Edinburgh Medical Journal* 45:605–619.

Cook, S. W. (1939) The Production of Experimental Neurosis in the White rat. *Psychosomatic Medicine* 1:293–308.

Dworkin, S., Baxt, J., and Dworkin, E. (1942) Behavioral Disturbance of Vomiting and Micturition in Conditioned Cats. *Psychosomatic Medicine* 4:75–81.

Gantt, W. H. (1944) *Experimental Basis for Neurotic Behavior*. Harper: New York.

Gantt, W. H. (1962) Factors Involved in the Development of Pathological Behavior: Schizokinesis and Autokinesis. *Perspectives in Biology and Medicine* 5:473–482.

Gantt, W. H. (1971) Experimental Basis for Neurotic Behavior. In *Experimental Psychopathology: Recent Research and Theory*, H. D. Kimmel, (Ed.). New York: Academic Press, pp. 33–47.

Hebb, D. O. (1947) Spontaneous Neurosis in Chimpanzees: Theoretical Relations With Clinical and Experimental Phenomena. *Psychosomatic Medicine* 9:3–16.

Kimmel, H. D. (Ed.) (1971) *Experimental Psychopathology: Recent Research and Theory*. New York: Academic Press.

Kubie, L. A. (1939) The Experimental Induction of Neurotic Reactions in Man. *Yale Journal of Biology and Medicine* 11:541–545.

Liddell, H. S. (1947) The Experimental Neurosis. Annual *Review of Physiology* IX: 569–580.

Liddell, H. S., and Bayne, T. L. (1927) The Development of Experimental Neurasthenia in the Sheep During the Formation of Difficult Conditioned Reflexes. *American Journal of Physiology* **81**:494–501.

Liddell, H. S., Anderson, O. D., Kotyuka, E., and Hartman, F. Z. (1935) The Effect of Extract of Adrenal Cortex on Experimental Neurosis in Sheep. *Archives of Neurology and Psychiatry* **34**:973–993.

Masserman, J. H. (1943) *Behavior and Neurosis: An Experimental Psychoanalytic Approach to Psychobiologic Principles.* Chicago: University of Chicago Press.

Masserman, J. H. (1961) *Principles of Dynamic Psychiatry.* Philadelphia: Saunders.

Masserman, J. H. (1971) The Principle of Uncertainty in Neurotigenesis. In *Experimental Psychopathology: Recent Research and Theory,* H. D. Kimmel (Ed.). New York: Academic Press.

Masserman, J. H., Arieff, A., Pechtel, C. and Kehr, H. (1950) Effects of Direct Interrupted Electroshock on Experimental Neurosis. *Journal of Nervous and Mental Disease* **112**:384–392.

Pavlov, I. P. (1928) *Lectures on Conditioned Reflexes.* New York: International Publishers.

Pavlov, I. P. (1941) *Lectures on Conditioned Reflexes: Vol. 2, Conditioned Reflexes and Psychiatry* (W. H. Gantt, trans.). New York: International Publishers.

Shenger-Krestovinikova, N. R. (1921) Contributions to the Questions of Differentiation of Visual Stimuli and the Limits of Differentiation by the Visual Analyzer of the Dog. *Bulletin of the Lesgaft Institute of Petrograd* (reference as given in Maser and Seligman, *Psychopathology: Experimental Models*).

Stainbrook, E. (1947) The Experimental Induction of Acute Animal Behavioral Disorders as a Method of Psychosomatic Research. *Psychosomatic Medicine* **9**:256–259.

Philosophical Basis for the Development of Animal Models for Psychiatric Illnesses

Introduction

This may be the most important chapter in this book. Though there is considerable activity and excitement in the animal modeling, or what might be called "comparative psychiatry," area, there is no conceptual framework for guiding the development of this field. The relevant basic sciences are scattered and have not been brought together in any organized manner as they relate to the development of animal models. We do not know how to evaluate proposed animal models for a given disorder or even how to conceptualize the roles for animal models as part of a spectrum of approaches in psychopathology research.

It is not that there is a total void of literature relevant to the above topics; but it is so scattered that it is functionally unavailable to most clinicians. Many examples are given in this chapter to illustrate this point, and a conceptual framework regarding animal models is proposed. It is hoped that this framework will be useful to both clinicians and basic researchers.

There are a variety of approaches to modeling, not all of which involve animals. Within the animal modeling area there are many approaches. Some focus on developmental and behavioral issues while others focus on neurobiological aspects. Some models are empirically developed to screen drugs while others are theoretically driven to evaluate etiological theories of psychopathology. None is comprehensive, and all have certain advantages and limitations. This chapter attempts to clarify some of these issues and to develop more realistic and appropriate expectations of animal modeling research.

One of the areas of often unspoken tension within psychiatry involves the interface between the "new neurobiology" and the social–developmental determinants of psychopathology. Each sphere has its strong and effective advocates, and the field of animal modeling research often gets caught up in these nonsensical debates. Perhaps the most important issue facing our field today is the development of appropriate, data-based conceptual models to account for the multiple variables that can lead to the development of psychopathology. Animal models have a role to play in this development, and this chapter tries to outline a beginning framework for their participation.

Some, including myself, have wondered if the term "animal models" should be dropped. It is so often poorly understood, controversial, and misused that a convincing case could be made to disband its use. However, I think the term is here to stay, so we should be clear as possible how we are using it and develop a framework for improving our multiple uses of the term. That is the primary intent of this chapter.

What Are Models?

The concept of "animal models" for psychiatric illnesses has become a controversial one, so perhaps some discussion of how the term should, and should not, be used is in order. As will be apparent in subsequent chapters when the approaches currently being used to develop animal models of different forms of psychopathology are described, the word is used in many different ways. Basically, animal models should be viewed as experimental preparations developed in one species for the purpose of studying phenomena occurring in another species. In the case of animal models of human psychopathology, one seeks to develop, in animals, syndromes which in certain ways resemble those in humans, in order to study selected aspects of the human psychopathology. Syndromes in animals will not resemble those in humans entirely. There will inevitably be important differences, and sometimes the study of these differences may be as important as the similarities.

Of course, animal models are experimentally induced and, surprisingly, have received a good deal of negative criticism because of this. They are viewed by some critics as artificial, nonspontaneous in origin, and, therefore, of little relevance to human psychopathology. However, within these objections lies a fundamental misunderstanding of human psychopathology. Most psychiatric illnesses do not arise *de novo*. There are vulnerabilities, causes, triggers, precipitants, etc. It is these, and their interactions, on which modern day animal modeling research focuses. The fact that an altered behavior is experimentally induced rather than naturally occuring does not make it any less valid. As a matter of fact, animal models are one way of evaluating, in a controlled manner, the effects of various possible inducing conditions.

There are a variety of approaches to modeling including computer simulation, mathemetical models, experimentally induced states in humans, and model neuronal systems in invertebrates. Some researchers, especially basic neuroscientists, in talking about animal models, equate them with the use of animals to contribute to our understanding of psychopathology by permitting direct study of the brain's functioning. A given model is evaluated by how well it lends itself to studies of underlying neurobiological mechansims by such techniques as single-unit recording, brain lesions, receptor studies, etc. With the rapid technological developments in the molecular neurosciences, animal models that lend themselves easily to these kinds of studies are currently in vogue. There is a strong tendency now to give highest priority to the development of animal models that will permit the utilization of many of the high-technology neuroscience techniques, and to de-emphasize the study of social behavior. The logic behind this approach seems to be very reductionistic in nature in that the proper study of behavior is conceptualized as the highly sophisticated study of neurons. While it is extremely important to continue to develop effective and meaningful systems in animals in which to do such studies, they are not the only kind of animal models. Other models make possible the more sophisticated and quantitative assessment of social behavior including the role of developmental and social inducing factors. This book gives examples of both kinds of experimental models under the specific disorders and presents the case for continuing to support the development of a plurality of experimental model systems, each with its own contributions and limitations.

There is no such thing as a comprehensive animal model for any psychiatric syndrome. However, if there were, under the most ideal of circumstances, an animal model of a specific illness would be identical to the human illness in terms of etiology, symptoms, underlying mechanisms, and treatment responsiveness. No such complete model exists for any psychiatric syndrome, nor is it likely that it will. There can only be successive approximations or simulations of specific, but limited, aspects of a given syndrome. However, there is much to be learned from a comparative approach in psychiatry, as there is in many fields of medicine, and the value of using animal models to study aspects of specific human syndromes is discussed later in this chapter as well as under the different syndromes. However, it is important to keep in mind that animal models are not replicas, nor do they represent the human illness in miniature. Historically, many approaches to animal modeling have made this mistake. As mentioned before, one characteristic of models is that they are different from the original illness or syndrome in some respects, and these differences may be as important to know about and study as the similarities.

Psychiatric illnesses are syndromes. Rarely do they have a single etiology but, rather, usually involve multiple variables interacting to account for different proportions of the variance in different individuals. Consequently, it is proving difficult to develop a data-based integrative view of most forms of human psychopathology. Such an integrative framework, based partly on animal work, has been described for human depression (Akiskal and McKinney, 1973, 1975; Klein, 1974; Whybrow, Akiskal, and McKinney, 1984; Whybrow and Parlatore, 1973). With multiple variables, each having main effects plus interactions, it becomes difficult on the basis of human clinical research alone to determine their relative influence. Animal models permit evaluation of the effects of these etiological variables one at a time and, in a systematic and controlled way, the nature of their interactions. Furthermore, from the standpoint of phenomenology, psychiatric syndromes involve a mixture of cognitive, emotional, affective, behavioral, and physiological manifestations. A model is an experimental preparation in which one or more of the symptoms or signs of the human syndrome is present and can be studied. As mentioned above, a model is not the reproduction of all the signs and symptoms of the illness in some replica form. This is an improper conceptualization of what models should be. Models should be designed along much more limited but useful grounds, such as to develop an experimental system in which to study a specific sign or symptom or to evaluate a specific etiological theory in a way that cannot be done in humans. Another possibility is to evaluate the effect of a specific treatment intervention on a particular behavior. This is quite different from the more frequent use of models, which is to use them for drug evaluation studies in a more global sense and to say a model is or is not valid on the basis of how clinically effective drugs work.

Arising out of the above reasoning, one can then speak of the following general kinds of animal models:

1. Behavioral similarity models: (those designed to simulate a specific sign or symptom of the human disorder).
2. Theory-driven models: (those designed to evaluate a specific etiological theory).
3. Mechanistic models: (those designed to study underlying mechanisms).
4. Empirical validity models: (those designed to permit preclinical drug evaluations).

General Kinds of Animal Models

Behavioral Similarity Models

In this approach to animal modeling ones tries to produce, in animals, certain specific aspects of the human disorder. The primary intent is not to evaluate either a specific etiological theory or treatment responsiveness. Obviously, these are important questions even in this kind of modeling but are not the primary focus. In this context, the validity of the model is judged by how closely it approximates the human condition. The reason for developing this kind of model is to focus on the study of a particular symptom or a cluster of symptoms. The methods used to induce the behavior may or may not be how such behaviors are produced in humans. An example could be given from outside psychiatry to illustrate this point. In the study of atherosclerosis in monkeys, the techniques that may be used to produce atherosclerotic blood vessels are, from one standpoint, secondary. The final common state, namely atherosclerosis, is the object of study. For example, a drug or a diet that is never used in humans may be used in animals to produce the state. Nevertheless, it may be a useful animal preparation in that a variety of mechanism studies and even treatment studies can be done. However, it would not be possible to make etiological statements from such studies.

Another example could be cited, this time from psychiatry. Stereotopy is a behavior that occurs in a number of psychiatic syndromes, and there are a number of ways to produce this behavior in animals.

(These are reviewed in more detail in the chapter on schizophrenia.) Several drugs can be used as well as social isolation or overcrowding. It may even be a trait-related characteristic of certain animals. This kind of animal preparation can then be used to further dissect stereotypic behaviors in a specific species. Since stereotypy is an important psychopathological behavior in humans with a variety of illnesses, such studies are potentially clinically relevant. However, it is not necessary to equate the stereotypic behavior being studied with any one specific clinical syndrome. Studies of the phenomena are important in their own right. More animal modeling work of just this kind needs to be done as part of an effort to develop general principles of psychopathology.

Theory-Driven Models

In this type of experimentation, we begin with a specific theory of a given form of psychopathology or, alternatively, with a general theory about the importance of certain variables in a number of forms of psychopathology. Typically, such theories have developed from studies of sick humans and, therefore, are retrospective in nature. This is an area where suitable animal preparations can play a particularly useful role. We can evaluate prospectively the effects of paradigms designed to represent certain causative theories. For example, clinical evidence suggests that separation is an important variable in the occurrence of certain types of depressions. This evidence, however, comes mostly from clinical retrospective studies and from population surveys. These are important sources of data, but it has generally been impossible in humans to evaluate prospectively the role of such separations and to what extent they were primary or derivative occurrences. That is, do people get depressed and then behave in ways that promote separations, or do the separations precede depression? What is the nature of their interaction? In animal preparations, one can study animals which have been subjected to controlled separations and prospectively evaluate the consequences. Such studies are worthwhile whether or not the state so induced in animals should properly be labeled depression. The induced state represents the use of animal preparations to test, in a systematic manner, the effects of certain inducing conditions, and permits the development of careful descriptions of the behavioral and neurobiological effects. Furthermore, how alterations in one or another parameter influence the response to a particular event can be quantified.

The use of animals in this way obviously involves the development of paradigms which reasonably simulate theories developed from clinical research. However, such experimental paradigms are available for a number of theories and are illustrated in subsequent chapters of this book. It should be emphasized that this use of animal models does not make any *a priori* assumptions about the validity of the theory. Rather, animal modeling researchers try to operationalize the theory and develop experimental paradigms to evaluate the effects of such inducing conditions. Modeling research has sometimes been unjustifiably criticized on the basis that the theory driving the development of the experimental paradigm has not been substantiated in humans. There is more than a touch of irony to this criticism because that is the very reason for developing the model in the first place, that is, to test the theory.

These "theory-driven" models are distinguished from the previous kind of model involving behavioral similarities that are more atheoretical. However, a key qualification is in order. These models are indeed theory driven in the sense that a theory drives the development of the paradigm; but they are not theory driven in the sense that one must assume the validity of the theory to value the research.

Mechanistic Models

Mechanistic models are at present a complex and controversial topic. To begin with, the topic involves a discussion of what is meant by "mechanisms." To some the term is synonomous with neurobiological mechanisms, and the value of animal models is directly related to how easily direct studies of such underlying mechanisms can be done. There are many examples of such approaches, mostly in invertebrates and rodents. Typically in such studies the description of behavior is quite limited. The neurobiological aspects will be very precise, but the behavioral descriptions either nonexistent or global.

To the developmentalist or the behaviorist "mechanism" might have very different meanings, and there would be much lower priority given to the development of animal preparations for study of central neurobiological mechanisms. Typically in such studies the behavioral descriptions, whether they be of social behavior or operant behavior, will be quite precise, but neurobiological indices minimally, if at all, assessed.

It is unfortunate that these approaches are developing in oppositional ways. They should be viewed as complementary. What often happens at present is that some approaches to animal modeling are criticized because they do not involve, or even permit, direct studies of underlying central mechanisms, whereas other approaches that pre-dominantly focus on central neurobiological mechanisms are criticized because they cannot, or do not, include descriptions of social behavior. There is room for both approaches. It is to be hoped that such antagonisms just represent a stage in the development of the field and will soon disappear.

In this day of high-technology neuroscience, it should not be forgotten that behavior and psychopathology occur in a social context, and therefore the continued study of social behavior is essential. On the other hand, not all kinds of animal preparations can permit satisfactory assessment of social behavior, but they may have other advantages. A very serious, indeed critical, challenge is the development of techniques to do mechanism studies in socially behaving animals. This may be the most important single challenge facing animal modeling researchers. On the one hand, there is an amazing array of techniques being developed to study central mechanisms of behavior down to the cellular and subcellular levels. On the other hand, the use of such techniques at present is limited to invertebrates, rodents, or chaired primates. This is not intended to disparage such studies, but there is a need to develop the next step, which is to study socially behaving higher-order animals in order to develop a richer understanding of the interaction of neurobiology and social behavior in psychopathology.

One cannot necessarily directly transpose techniques of mechanism studies from rodents to monkeys or, for that matter, from monkeys to humans. The study of mechanisms must be approached from different vantage points in different species and in different protocols. Each approach has advantages and disadvantages. The appropriateness of each technique must be evaluated on a number of grounds including species, economics, ethics, the kind of behavioral data desired, etc. Additional detail regarding the use of animal models for mechanism studies is given under each syndrome.

Empirical Validity Models

If we are mainly interested in developing an animal model system in which drugs can be evaluated, the method of inducing the syndrome and even the behavioral similarity issues become secondary. We then evaluate the animal model by how well the effects of the drug in question in the model predict clinical effects or, conversely, how well drugs that work in humans also work in the model. This is called empirical validity, and a number of approaches to animal modeling have this as their major goal. A number of useful models that have empirical validity are available in psychiatry and have been particularly important in the advancement of psychopharmacology. However, this does not necessarily mean that the model in question has anything to do with the human syndrome. The empirical validity of a model does not establish it as valid on other grounds. For example, drugs may work in a given animal model and predict clinical effectiveness quite well. However, drugs may have the same effects in two species for quite different reasons. The fact that the ability of a given drug to prevent reserpine-induced sedation is correlated with its effectiveness as a clinical antidepressant does not necessarily establish reserpine-induced sedation as a valid animal model of depression. Validity is a relative concept and has to be considered in relationship to the reasons for the development of the model in the first place. This stipulation does not make the reserpine-induced sedation model, or any other model with high empirical validity, any less important, but it does circumscribe the kinds of conclusions that can be drawn from the model.

This use of models represents one of the oldest and most widely known. The pharmaceutical industry has pioneered in the development of such models. In an ideal model there should be no false positives and no false negatives. That is, in all instances a drug that works in the animal model should also work clinically in humans and vice versa. This goal has never been achieved nor is it likely that it will, although there are a number of paradigms which have high empirical validity for depression, schizophrenia, and anxiety.

The Homology–Analogy Issue

Another controversial issue which frequently arises in discussion of animal models is the question of whether a given model is homologous or analogous. Homology assumes both similarity in function and commonality in evolutionary mechanisms. Thus, homologous models, almost by definition, are a theoretical construct, unavailable for any clinical psychiatric syndrome. Therefore it is an unreasonable requirement to insist that they are the only appropriate models. They would have the advantage that the assumption could be made that what is learned from one species (the model) can be directly applied to another species (the modeled). However, even if we tried to defend a given model as homologous, it would be difficult to establish that the phenomenon was not significantly influenced by processes of evolutionary divergence. The issue is even more complicated. As Eibl-Eibesfeldt says, "when we speak of homologies, we generally attribute shared characteristics to common genetic heritage" (1983, p. 51). Wickler (1965) distinguishes between phyletic homologies and homologies of tradition. According to Wickler, homology indicates that, underlying the patterns in question, only a common source of information was tapped. Whether this information has been stored in the genome or as cultural knowledge is left open.

Curiously enough, some animal models are criticized for being only analogous rather than homologous. This criticism generally reflects an ignorance of the ethological and evolutionary literature. It would be very difficult to defend any behavioral model as homologous, but this does not mean the model is any less useful. Analogous models assume only common function and not necessarily common ancestry or mechanisms. The advantage of analogous models is that functional behaviors can be compared in species that have undergone convergent evolution, and the behavior being compared need not be similar in form or in underlying mechanisms—just similar in function. Again to quote Eibl-Eibesfeldt:

> the study of analogous development certainly allows us to develop hypotheses about the advantages of certain behavior which then have to be tested in each special case. This holds true in general for the comparative approach. We never make any immediate inferences from the study of geese or fish as to rules governing human behavior, but we develop hypotheses that guide our attention, which in each case have to be tested by the study of man. (1983, p. 47)

The disadvantage of analogous models is that a behavior which serves a certain function in one species might serve other functions in other species. Also, what is learned about mechanisms in one species may not necessarily be the same mechanisms underlying similar behaviors in another species.

Neither type of model is inherently good or bad. Both have their advantages and limitations, and the most important issue is that the investigator recognizes these in the design of experiments and in the interpretation of data. The view that only homologies count is mistaken. While it is true that analogies tell us something different from homologies, both have their place. And finally to quote Eibl-Eibesfeldt:

> . . . for those interested in the evolution of particular structures, homologies are the focal point of interest. The study of analogies, on the other hand, informs us about the selection pressures that shaped these structures and caused processes of behavior to develop along similar lines. In fact, the laws found by the study of analogies are of wider applicability, and thus more general and fundamental than those discovered by the study of homol-

ogues. Should one, therefore, be interested in phenomena like ranking, territoriality, or mating systems, it is certainly advisable to study these in many different groups of animals, regardless of their phylogenetic relationship. The further apart they are, the better, because only then can we be sure that the regularities observed can be attributed to the more general laws of function and not derived from a genetic relationship. (1983, p. 44)

Why Have Animal Models?

As was pointed out by Abramson and Seligman (1977), the development of animal models has played an important role in the evolution of the field of psychopathology from case history, observation, and speculation, to a controlled setting in which a particular symptom or constellation of symptoms is produced in order to explicitly test hypotheses about cause and cure. The logic behind modeling is that by examining the model we can learn more about the etiology, cure, and prevention of the naturally occurring psychopathology.

Many of the critical questions about human psychopathology cannot be studied in humans, but if appropriate animal models can be developed, such questions can be addressed. For example, prospective studies examining the effects of developmental events on behavior and on neurochemistry can be done within the lifetime of an investigator studying animals. The interaction between variables can be studied in a controlled manner. There are animal preparations which have been developing in the last decade which make such investigations feasible and will facilitate the movement beyond correlation to cause-and-effect studies.

Studies of human psychiatric illnesses have historically started at the time of the event and worked backward through the use of diagnosis and recollection. Obviously we cannot attempt to produce psychological aberrations in patients. Ethical and practical considerations also prevent the control of certain key variables. Through the use of animal models it is possible to control environmental boundaries, arrange case histories, produce severe syndromes, and experiment with untested drugs and combinations of drugs.

Animal models potentially make possible the dissection of underlying mechanisms in a more direct way than is possible in human clinical research but complement ongoing efforts in this regard. Attention needs to be paid to how to do what kind of mechanism studies in a given species, but this is a major reason for developing animal models.

Animal Modeling Research in Relationship to Other Approaches in Psychiatric Research

Before proceeding to a discussion of the evaluation of animal models, it may be helpful to consider the rationale for models and their role in a spectrum of approaches to psychiatric research. In this context, some additional contributions which animal models can make are given along with their limitations.

Historically, psychiatry has relied heavily on case histories in its theory development. Starting with a sick population, etiological theories have evolved in the process of treatment. Such theories have provided us with a framework for understanding psychopathology, but since the development of such theories has been based on retrospective data obtained from sick patients and/or relatives, their general validity has been suspect.

The limitations of this approach have long been recognized, and other research methods have been sought. Another approach, epidemiological in nature, involved various types of community sampling techniques. In more recent years there has been increased clinical research activity in controlled settings. Patients with specified diagnoses are carefully studied with highly developed neurobiological techniques and behaviorally assessed with many rating scales. Patients are studied longitudinally through the course of their illnesses.

The special contribution of animal modeling research to this spectrum of psychiatric research activity is in the ability to control the inducing condition and study the behavioral and biological effects on both a short- and long-term basis. Furthermore, the nature of the interaction among developmental, social, and biological variables in a social species can be studied in a meaningful way. In human clinical research, multiple variables interact simultaneously, and it is typically impossible to sort out these variables in any quantifiable way. It is at this interface that animal modeling research has a unique contribution to make. In animal studies the precise inducing condition is known, and other variables can be kept constant.

Until recently animal modeling research was not taken seriously by psychiatrists. Some of the reasons for this are historical and result from a far too vague use of clinical terms and the use of inducing procedures which were foreign to most psychiatrists. The situation has now changed within the animal modeling field in that there are some useful animal preparations for studying important questions about human psychopathology. These are illustrated in subsequent chapters.

Limitations of Animal Models

There are limitations in the use of animal models that must be recognized and considered in the interpretation of data. Perhaps the main one concerns cross-species reasoning difficulties. While it is true that certain animal species have many behavioral and physical traits in common with humans, there are differences, and one cannot reason directly from the results in one species to another. Not all species, even those which are phylogenetically very close, necessarily respond in the same fashion, or even in the same intensity, to identical events or stimulations. This is exemplified in the research of Kaufman and Rosenblum (1967a, 1967b; Rosenblum and Kaufman, 1968) with pigtail (*Macaca nemestrina*) and bonnet (*Macaca radiata*) monkeys. When the mothers of young pigtails were removed from the established troop, the youngsters went into a decline, evincing signs of "despair" or "depression." The infant bonnets in the same situation did not show any of these signs. This difference might be explained by differences in the social structure of the two species. Adult female bonnets and their infants spend a lot of time in social contact with one another, while adult female pigtails and their infants are very much "dyadic loners." As a result, the infant bonnets had stabilized relationships both with other adults and other infants to draw on when their mothers were removed. This was not the case with the pigtail infants. If, however, young bonnets lost the supporting members of their troop, they might show the same behavioral traits as the pigtail infants. There would then be a situation in which the primary inducing cause (loss of an important affectional object) was similar, but the actual event was different. With increased study and information, these differences can be accounted for and integrated into the various theories of behavior.

A very important way in which the study of animal behavior can aid in the understanding of human behavior is in the description and classification of behaviors. Ethologists have contributed to the careful dissection and description of behavior into its component parts including the context in which the behavior occurs. Psychiatrists and comparative psychologists have begun considering this issue again. We have become very descriptive with the criteria for our diagnoses. Animal behavior research can help sensitize us in this area and help with the development of improved observational techniques. For example, there are a number of highly sophisticated behavioral scoring systems for describing animals' social behavior in the field, in seminaturalistic settings, and in the laboratory. Such parameters as duration, frequency, sequence, and reciprocity can be quantified. These techniques have only rarely been used to study psychiatric patients, even though most major forms of psychopathology involve significant alterations in behavior and in patterns of social relationships.

We must be content with utilizing generalizations of limited scope. This concept was best expressed by Hinde, who wrote, "The scope of any generalization is inversely related to its precision" (1972, p. 12). As more behaviors are lumped together in broader categories, sensitivity to precise, limited occurrences is lost. If we can avoid this tendency, our ability to make cross-species guesses will be greatly enhanced. Ultimately, we will have to develop hypotheses based on experimental work with animals and test them directly in humans, rather than reasoning directly from results in one species to another.

Often in this area we are talking about the establishment of principles of animal behavior and assessment of their applicability to humans, that is, the overlapping territories of psychiatry and ethology (Grant, 1965; Hutt, 1970; Jones, 1971; Kraemer, 1977; Lehrman, 1974; McGuire and Fairbanks, 1977; Zegans, 1967). This is an area where the study of animal behavior can be a special asset. While we should in no way dismiss or underestimate the complexity of interactions in animals, we can, nevertheless, isolate behaviors and sets of behaviors and study them in a more controlled manner than can be done in humans. As a result, it is possible to highlight certain theoretical issues. This can be an especially dangerous procedure and has been grossly misused by certain writers who, by selecting facts to fit preconceived theories and neglecting awkward cases, have tried to take a very reductionistic view of human behavior. However, with caution and concern, this snare can be circumvented and does not negate the value of the above principle properly used in assessing human behavior.

Humans and their fellow primates are alike in many aspects of social behavior and physical structure. Research into animal behavior that is tempered by an awareness and consideration of not only those traits which are similar but also of those which are unique to either may provide new information and understanding of the model. This in turn may provide a more accurate means by which human behavior can be assessed and interpreted.

Evaluation of Animal Models

How does one evaluate animal models? Several investigators have written on this subject (Abramson and Seligman, 1977; Hamburg, 1968;

Ingle and Shein, 1975; Kormetsky, 1977; Levy, 1952; McKinney and Bunney, 1969; Mitchel, 1970; Serban and Kling, 1976; Startsev, 1976; Suomi and Immelman, 1983; Zubin and Hunt, 1967). The present section draws on many of these contributions but also tries to discuss the question of evaluation in a different framework from those presented previously.

The evaluation of an animal model should closely relate to the purposes for which the model is being developed in the first place. To cite an extreme example, a model created to screen for antidepressant drugs may have high empirical validity in that context but be completely inappropriate for studying various etiological theories. On the other hand a model developed to evaluate a given etiological variable in depression might be completely inappropriate or impractical for drug screening. It is not a matter of one kind of modeling approach being better or worse. It is a question of why the model is being developed in the first place and how it is to be used. Investigators need to be clear on this point. It is no longer possible, and probably never was, to think of a comprehensive model for any one clinical syndrome.

Abramson and Seligman (1977) point out that it is important to know the "essential" features of the model. They cite the example of inescapable electric shock. If shock itself were the important variable, then the paradigm would be relevant only to the production of psychopathology in concentration camps or other such places. On the other hand, if the shock is just a tool to induce a given state, and the issue is uncontrollable aversive events in general, then the paradigm has far-reaching significance for human psychopathology.

Other examples of this very important principle could be given. Amphetamine is known to induce stereotypic behaviors and other changes in animals. How relevant and generalizable is this as a schizophrenia model? If amphetamine is necessary to produce the stereotypy, the model may be relevant only to amphetamine or similar drug-induced states in humans. However, if amphetamine should prove to be one of several tools, all of which induce similar neurochemical changes, then these changes may be the essential features and the paradigm may be important for studying the connection between this set of neurochemical changes and a particular behavior which can occur in schizophrenia. On the other hand, the neurochemical substrates may be a less important aspect of this model. The model may be more useful as a screen for neuroleptic drugs. In this sense the model may have empirical validity without necessarily having anything to do with human schizophrenia.

Another example of this principle is the separation paradigm in monkeys. Separation is a tool for inducing a specified set of behavioral and physiological changes, some of which are characteristic of some human depressions and which can be studied in animal preparations. Similar changes can be induced by other methods, which makes the behaviors even more important to study and suggests that the changes have some more generalized significance. The importance of the paradigm does not rest on whether or not separations cause human depressions. Alone, they clearly do not, although the evidence is very strong that they are important risk factors. The main point about animal models is that they are a means to an end.

We and others have previously proposed that one criterion to use in evaluating animal models involves similarity of inducing conditions. That is, a given animal paradigm is or is not valid to the extent that the condition used to produce the animal preparation is also operative in humans with that illness. There is a problem with this criterion. There are no forms of human psychopathology for which a specific etiology is known to the extent that it can be used as a necessary criterion in animal modeling studies. However, we are learning new things about risk factors for some illnesses, and the continued development of paradigms in which to evaluate these risk factors would be an important contribution of animal models.

While we do not know enough about the etiology of any form of psychopathology to use this as a necessary or validating criterion for a given animal model, the inducing techniques which are used in animal modeling research should bear a reasonably close relationship to variables thought to be important in human psychopathology. This does not mean that we should use only inducing techniques whose causative association with a human syndrome has been clearly established, but there should be an attempt to relate closely to ongoing clinical research and to complement such research by doing prospective and controlled evaluations of theories. As more carefully controlled studies in humans become available, there will be a broader data base for the development of animal paradigms than there has been previously.

Another proposed method for evaluating animal models is the requirement that they have the same underlying mechanisms as the human syndrome being modeled. This includes such things as a similar physiology or neurobiology. This criterion, while correct in theory, is impractical. There is no known neurobiological change for any form of human psychopathology that we could say must be present in a given animal model for that model to be valid on this ground. In other words, the mechanisms criterion cannot at present be necessary, but it must be considered in relationship to a number of other aspects of the model.

Animal models should be developed with a major purpose being to study underlying mechanisms in a way not possible in humans, but, as previously discussed, it is important to plan carefully since the type of mechanism study that is important to do in rodents, for example, may not be indicated in primates where one is also studying social behavior.

In evaluating animal models, it should be kept in mind that some may model specific aspects of certain clinical disorders, whereas others may model some fundamental features that are important for many forms of psychopathology. There is a need for models in both of these areas, and it should not always be necessary to anchor the research to a specific syndrome. There is increasing pressure to do this, but in the long run it is shortsighted.

An additional way in which animal models are frequently evaluated regards their responsiveness to pharmacological agents. A given animal model is said to be valid or not valid to the extent that it is influenced by pharmacological agents in a like manner as in humans. For example, stereotypic behaviors produced by amphetamine and certain other drugs have been proposed as an animal model of schizophrenia largely on the basis of the response of such behaviors to pharmacological agents. Drugs which are effective in treating human schizophrenia also reverse the stereotypic behaviors in animals, and drugs which are ineffective clinically do not. Likewise, reserpine-induced hypothermia, ptosis, and other changes seen in rodents have been presented as an animal model of depression because clinically effective antidepressants prevent this syndrome. There are many other examples, since this method of empirically evaluating animal models has been widely used. We could develop for each animal preparation a profile of pharmacological responsiveness. In general, clinically effective drugs should work, but ineffective ones should not. However, a word of caution is in order when evaluating models by this criterion. There is no perfect match in this regard. There are always false positives and false negatives. There will inevitably be clinically effective drugs which will not work in a given animal model and situations in which a drug will work in a given animal model but be completely ineffective in humans. We cannot make definitive statements about the validity of a given model solely on the basis of its response to drugs. This is not surprising given possible species differences in the metabolism and neurobiological effects of drugs. These data must be considered in relationship to all the other methods for evaluating models. Similarity of drug response across species thus is neither a necessary nor sufficient criterion.

How then are we to evaluate models? The task isn't easy because there are no absolute standards other than very idealistic ones. To quote Hanin and Usdin (1977):

> A good animal model of any particular disease state is one which will simulate and reproduce most accurately the human syndrome which it is designed to represent. Ideally it should mirror behaviorally the symptoms of the disorder and should respond to pharmacologic and appropriate therapeutic agents in a manner identical to that observed in the original human state. (p. XIII)

I could add to the above goal the concept of studying mechanisms and the ability of the model to facilitate such studies. I doubt that this utopian goal will ever be achieved in any one model.

In reality there is room and need for a plurality of animal models for a given psychiatric illness. There is no "best" model for any syndrome. Basically, the investigator should have done as thorough an experimental analysis of the model as possible so that the critical features can be described. The focus may be on a specific response, whether it is behavioral, electrophysiological, or neurochemical, and on how this response is affected by interventions used in the treatment of certain human syndromes. The induction techniques used to produce these responses may vary and all be worthy of study without having to necessarily be identical to the etiology of human disorders. This is especially true since in humans we often don't know the exact etiology. Until clinical research with humans pinpoints more specific etiologies, there is room for a variety of approaches in animal studies with regard to induction techniques. Such work may, as a matter of fact, lead to the development of improved etiological theories of clinical syndromes.

There is room and need for animal modeling studies in a variety of species. What species is appropriate depends on the questions being investigated, and there is a need to continue to develop different kinds of models in many species.

In summary, there is no universally valid model for any psychiatric syndrome. Instead, there are animal preparations available for studying specific aspects of a number of syndromes. The present state of affairs represents a significant improvement from the days when we thought there were some firm criteria by which to evaluate models and there was the search for the best model of a given syndrome. There are idealistic criteria but these must be applied with caution depending on the function of the particular model. I hope this represents evolution of the field and a more realistic assessment of its contributions, potential, and limitations than has sometimes been present. I also hope the remaining chapters in this book illustrate this philosophy in the context of specific psychiatric illnesses.

Summary of Key Points

- *Animal models are experimental preparations developed in one species for the purpose of studying phenomena occurring in another species.*

- *There is no such thing as a comprehensive animal model for any psychiatric syndrome nor will there ever be. Animal models should be designed and developed along more limited lines to study specific issues about human psychopathological syndromes.*

- *There are at least four different kinds of animals models, each with different purposes. They include (a) those designed to simulate specific signs or symptoms of a disorder, (b) those designed to evaluate specific etiological theories, (c) those designed to study underlying mechanisms, and (d) those designed to permit preclinical drug evaluations.*

- *A major reason for developing animal models is to study the interaction among variables in prospective studies and assist in moving clinical psychiatry away from deterministic views of the origins of psychopathology and toward an integrative view.*

- *The limitations of animal models must be recognized and dealt with. These mainly involve cross-species reasoning difficulties which can sometimes lead to excessive anthropomorphizing or, at other times, to total rejection of animal studies as irrelevant to human psychopathology.*

- *The evaluation of an animal model must relate closely to the purposes for which the model was developed in the first place. Arguments about which is the "best" model for a given syndrome are meaningless. It depends on what one wants to investigate in a given experimental paradigm. There is no such thing as a universally valid model for any syndrome, but there are animal preparations available for studying specific aspects of a number of syndromes. We very much need such a plurality of models and need to stop the search for the nonexistent complete model.*

References

Abramson, L. Y., and Seligman, M. (1977) *Psychopathology: Experimental Methods.* San Francisco: Freeman.

Akiskal, H. S., and McKinney, W. T. (1973) Depressive Disorders: Toward a Unified Hypothesis" *Science* **182**:20–29.

Akiskal, H. S., and McKinney, W. T. (1975) Overview of Recent Research in Depression: Integration of Ten Conceptual Models Into a Comprehensive Clinical Frame. *Archives of General Psychiatry* **32**:285–305.

Eibl-Eibesfeldt (1983) The Comparative Approach in Human Ethology. In *Comparing Behavior: Studying Man Studying Animals*, D. W. Rajecki (Ed.). Hillsdale, New Jersey: Lawrence Erlbaum.

Grant, E. C. (1965) The Contribution of Ethology to Child Psychiatry. In *Modern Perspectives in Child Psychiatry*, J. G. Howells (Ed.). Edinburgh: Oliver and Boyd.

Hamburg, D. A. (1968) Evolution of Emotional Responses: Evidence From Recent Research on Nonhuman Primates in *Science and Psychoanalysis: Vol. 12, Animal and Human*, J. H. Masserman (Ed.). New York: Grune and Stratton.

Hanin, I., and Usdin, E. (Eds.) (1977) *Animal Models in Psychiatry and Neurology*. Oxford: Pergamon Press.

Hinde, R. A. (1972) *Social Behavior and Its Development in Subhuman Primates*. Eugene, Oregon: Oregon State System of Higher Education.

Hutt, S. J. (1970) The Role of Behavior Studies in Psychiatry: an Ethological Viewpoint. In *Behavior Studies in Psychiatry*, S. J. Hutt and C. Hutt (Eds.). New York: Pergamon Press.

Ingle, D., and Shein, H. M. (Eds.) (1975) *Model systems in Biological Psychiatry*. Cambridge, Massachusetts: MIT Press.

Jones, I. H. (1971) Ethology and Psychiatry. *Australian and New Zealand Journal of Psychiatry* 5:258–263.

Kaufman, I. C., and Rosenblum, L. A. (1967a) The Reaction to Separation in Infant Monkeys: Anaclitic Depression and Conservation Withdrawal. *Psychosomatic Medicine* 29:648–675.

Kaufman, I. C., and Rosenblum, L. A. (1967b) Depression in Infant Monkeys Separated From Their Mothers. *Science* 155:1030–1031.

Klein, D. (1974) Endogenomorphic Depression: A Conceptual and Terminological Revision. *Archives of General Psychiatry* 31:447–454.

Kormetsky, C. (1977) Animal Models: Promises and Problems. In *Animal Models in Psychiatry and Neurology*, I. Hanin and E. Usdin (Eds.). New York: Pergamon.

Kraemer, S. (1977) Ethological Contributions to the Medical and Behavioral Sciences. In *The Future of Animals, Cells, Models, and Systems in Research, Development, Education, and Testing* Washington, D.C.: National Academy of Sciences.

Lehrman, D. S. (1974) Can Psychiatrists Use Ethology. In *Ethology and Psychiatry*, N. F. White (Ed.). Toronto: University of Toronto Press.

Levy, D. M. (1952) Animal Psychology in its Relation to Psychiatry. In *Dynamic Psychiatry* Franz Alexander and Helen Ross (Eds.). Chicago: University of Chicago Press.

McGuire, M. T., and Fairbanks, L. A. (1977) Ethology: Psychiatry's Bridge to Behavior. In *Ethological Psychiatry*, M. T. McGuire and L. A. Fairbanks (Eds.). New York: Grune and Stratton.

McKinney, W. T., and Bunney, W. E. (1969) Animal Model of Depression, Review of Evidence: Implications for Research. *Archives of General Psychiatry* 21:240–248.

Mitchell, G. D. (1970) Abnormal Behavior in Primates. In *Primate Behavior*, L. Rosenblum (Ed.). New York: Academic Press.

Rosenblum, L. A., and Kaufman, I. C. (1968) Variations in Infant Development and Response to Maternal Loss in Monkeys. *American Journal of Orthopsychiatry* 83:418–426.

Serban, G., and Kling, A. (Eds.) (1976) *Animal Models in Human Psychobiology*. New York: Plenum.

Startsev, V. G. (1976) *Primate Models of Human Neurogenic Disorders* (English translation edited by D. M. Bowden). Hillsdale, New Jersey: Lawrence Erlbaum.

Suomi, S. J., and Immelman, K. (1983) On the Process and Product of Cross- Species

Generalization. In *Comparing Behavior: Studying Man Studying Animals*. D. W. Rajecki (Ed.). Hillsdale, New Jersey: Lawrence Erlbaum.

Whybrow, P., Akiskal, H., McKinney, W. (1984) *Mood Disorders: Toward a New Psychobiology*. Plenum: New York.

Whybrow, P., and Parlatore, A. (1973) Melancholia: A Model in Madness: A Discussion of Recent Psychobiologic Research Into Depressive Illness. *International Journal of Psychiatry in Medicine* **4**:351–378.

Wickler, W. (1965) Uber den taxonomischen Wert Homologer Verhaltensmerkmale. *Naturwissenschaften* **52**:44–444.

Zegans, L. S. (1967) An Appraisal of Ethological Contributions to Psychiatric Theory and Research. *American Journal of Psychiatry* **124**:729–739.

Zubin, J., and Hunt, H. F. (Eds.) (1967) *Comparative Psychopathology: Animal and Human*. New York: Grune and Stratton.

II

Four Illustrative Case Examples

3

Animal Models for Affective Disorders

Introduction

This chapter begins the second section of the book, which is organized around four case examples, or illustrations, of psychopathological syndromes for which animal models have been proposed. The four clinical syndromes covered are affective disorders, anxiety disorders, schizophrenia, and alcoholism.

In this chapter, the animal modeling work relevant to affective disorders is reviewed in the context of the philosophical and historical perspectives previously provided. From the standpoint of sheer volume of publications and work, this is the largest research area. Furthermore, the biggest percentage of work relevant to animal modeling of affective disorders has been with depression rather than mania. There is a small, but significant, literature about the latter and this is discussed in this chapter.

The reader of this chapter will realize that there have been a very large number of animal models of depression proposed. Each has its effective advocates and critics. The general tendency has been to develop a given "model" and then to argue how it was the "best" animal model of depression. This enthusiasm has typically been countered by critics who point to the shortcomings of the model, and the literature multiplies exponentially. A certain amount of this has been healthy for the field and has led to scientific advances much as such interchanges often do in any field of science. However, to a certain extent, the development of the field has been hampered by these contentious exchanges.

The issue isn't which model is best but, rather, what questions can be addressed in a given experiment paradigm and which cannot. This involves being clear about the kind of model being developed and what its advantages and limitations are, given that no model will ever be a truly comprehensive one. Some are good for certain kinds of studies but not others. The field is now at a stage where this conceptualization is being slowly adopted, and the future thereby looks brighter.

It is sometimes said that the depression syndrome is easier to model in animals because of the availability of behavioral indices by which to measure it. To a certain extent this may be true, but there are many kinds of depressions, and one has to guard against a tendency to prematurely apply a clinical label to animals' behavior in this area. The clinician, in reading this chapter, will see that many constellations of behavioral changes resulting from different inducing conditions are sometimes labeled depression. Care needs to be exercised, and the differences among the kinds of models and ways to evaluate them, as discussed in previous chapters, should be kept in mind. There is an attempt to help the reader with this as the different approaches to modeling are reviewed.

Though representative models are presented, and there is a deliberate attempt to be broad, one cannot be all-inclusive in a book of this size. For example, this chapter on affective disorders could be expanded to a book (or several books) by itself. The review of the proposed models is also not intended to be comprehensive; rather it is an introduction designed to illustrate some of the general points made earlier. This means that, by and large, original data are not presented. These data are available in the referenced journals. It also means that the most recent data in a given area is not necessarily presented. A book-type format is not the best place to do this, as the information would likely be outdated by the time of publication.

History

The history of animal modeling research in depression dates back to at least 1928, with the earliest stage consisting largely of case reports. For example, Tinkelpaugh (1928) reported the case of Cupid, a young, male rhesus monkey who developed marked behavioral changes including self-mutilation, agitation, anorexia, and social withdrawal following separation and subsequent viewing of a female monkey with whom he had lived monogamously for 3 years. After reunion with the female, he gradually recovered. Yerkes and Yerkes (1929) wrote about the high death rate of newly captured gorillas and attributed this to "psychogenic" factors, citing the loss of familiar surroundings and the severance of all meaningful bonds as antecedent causes of their deaths. They also observed behavioral changes resembling depression in chimpanzees and suggested separation as a probable cause.

In addition to the above case reports, a number of other scattered reports suggested that a variety of animals might experience something akin to human depression. For example, Hebb (1947) reported the case of the chimpanzee Kambi, a wild-born animal raised in the lab with other chimpanzees during the early developmental period. She was noted to be "unpredictable, emotionally unstable, and introverted at maturity. Subsequently, during the postadolescent period she would have periodic episodes in which she would sit for hours with her back to the wall, staring at the floor of the cage and being unresponsive to other animals or to caretakers. Indeed, she was so unresponsive that she would not eat unless housed alone. These periods would last 6–8 months at a time, and between episodes she would appear well adjusted. The episodes could not be related to any specific events. She eventually died from dysentery while she was behaviorally abnormal.

These kinds of reports have continued to the present. Indeed, a veritable collection of such case histories could be assembled. They are available in abundance from the veterinary and medical literature as well as from such sources as veterinarians, keepers of kennels and pounds, zoos, primate research centers, and field studies.

Some may have found the above kinds of reports interesting, but the more serious development of the animal modeling field did not begin until there were controlled experimental methods of inducing such depressive-like syndromes. This is understandable because the technique of case collection could, and can, be done more easily in humans. The controlled production and experimental study of psychopathological states cannot be.

Several lines of research activity in the 1960s are relevant to the history of the experimental area of animal modeling. A study done by Senay (1966) represents one of the first explicit attempts to experimentally study depression in animals. In this study, the investigator himself formed a special relationship with each of a litter of 3-week-old German shepherd puppies over a 9-month period. During this time, he was their sole consistent human contact. Then, for a 2-month separation period, the animals had no contact with him. This was followed by a 1-month reunion period in which Senay resumed his former relationship with the animals. Independent observers gathered data on the animals' object-seeking, object-avoiding, and aggressive behaviors throughout the experiment. It was found that separation produced increases in object-seeking behavior for animals of the approach temperament, and increases in object avoidance and aggressive behavior for animals of the avoidance temperament. Senay thought that the observations supported the contention that animals exhibit predictable behavioral changes following object loss and indicated that experimental psycho-biological models of separation could be constructed in animals. Different animals react differently to attachment bond disruption, and special attention was called to the importance of temperament and the preloss levels of gratification in understanding separation phenomena.

Several other historical developments in this field should be mentioned. One is the development of separation paradigms, mainly in primates. The details of this approach are covered later in this chapter, but it is of interest that several laboratories, more or less independently, began a series of studies about separation of nonhuman primates, mostly of mothers and infants. These studies, begun in the 1960s and continuing to the present, have provided a considerable amount of data about the development and disruption of attachment bonds. There continues to be controversy about these studies, and all other approaches, regarding their validity as animal models of human depression, but it is argued throughout this chapter that each of these lines of work has merit *per se* apart from any possible linkage with human depression.

Another important line of work begun in the 1960s was the learned helplessness approach. This too is reviewed later in this chapter, but it is an approach which has spawned an enormous literature and relates closely to cognitive and, probably, neurobiological theories regarding human depression. From a theoretical standpoint, the learned helplessness and separation models are potentially closely linked in that the phenomenon of uncontrollability may be an important mediating variable in explaining the reactions to separation. Additional work is needed to investigate this possibility and to relate this possible mechanism to what is now known about the behavioral and neurobiological aspects of separation.

During the time that behavioral models of depression were being pursued, the development of pharmacological models for depression also continued. These too are the subject for a subsequent section of this chapter.

A fourth development in the animal modeling of depression area has involved the relationship among multiple stressors, conflict, and depression. Recently, animal paradigms have been developed for studying these interrelationships, and these paradigms provide a potentially important new development. They are also described later in this chapter.

Another type of approach to animal modeling of depression relates to alteration of dominance patterns. Several writers have speculated about the importance of such patterns in relationship to depression, though only limited empirical data are available.

As should be apparent from this brief review, there has been considerable evolution in the development of animal models of depression. The field has gone from early case histories to multiple experimental induction techniques. A variety of methods are currently used to develop new animal models of depression, and additional ones will continue to be developed. It should be emphasized that the field of animal models for depression is a relatively new one. At most, it has been in existence about 20 years, with most of the developments and advances occurring recently. There have been and will continue to be some false starts, but the field is progressing and is in a formative and exciting stage.

Clinical Considerations

It would not be possible in this section to provide a thorough clinical discussion of the depressive illnesses. This topic has already been the subject of countless books and articles. Rather, the focus is on those clinical considerations which are especially relevant for the development of animal models.

The first issue concerns the terms *endogenous* and *reactive* depression. The continued use of these or similar terms is distressing. They are widely used to distinguish between those depressions which arise from "within," without external causes and are heavily genetically and biologically based, from those depressions which occur in reaction to life events and are commonly thought more minor. This distinction is simply not supported by available data (Whybrow, Akiskal, and McKinney, 1984). The kind of symptom pattern in depression is relatively independent of the presence or absence of precipitants. That is, the person with an endogenous symptom pattern is just as likely (or unlikely) to have had a stressful event precede the depressive episode as is a person with a different kind of symptom pattern. In this context the original use of the terms *reactive* and *endogenous* needs to be remembered. They were originally introduced to describe the states of the depressed persons in terms of whether or not they were reactive to various inputs. The terms were not intended to have etiological meanings such as whether or not there were precipitants.

Attempts to develop animal models of depression have often been criticized because they are not spontaneous but, rather, follow some experimental induction technique. This nonspontaneity is contrasted to serious (or major) human depressions that allegedly occur spontaneously. An extension of this criticism has sometimes taken the form which can be paraphrased as the following: the model is relevant to only reactive depressions since something experimental was done to the animals to get them to behave in the way they are.

A more useful way to conceptualize human depressions is as a psychobiological final common pathway with numerous variables influencing whether or not depressions develop as well as the form of the depression. The details of this theory have been developed in several publications (Akiskal and McKinney, 1973, 1975; Whybrow and Parlatore, 1973; Whybrow et al., 1984). Basically, depressive illnesses are viewed as the culmination of various processes that influence brain function—probably diencephalic—and lead to changes in arousal, mood, cognition, psychomotor function, social behavior, etc. These processes include a number of variables, each of which can exert main effects but many of which certainly interact. A critical question in studying the etiology of most depressions is not what caused them but what proportion of the variance in their occurrence is accounted for by a series of interacting variables. These include, among others, genetic vulnerability, developmental events, interpersonal stressors, physiological stressors, and personality traits. There are theoretical models in many of these areas and empirical support for the involvement of many of them.

Given such a complex and multivariate illness, it becomes especially important to have experimental systems in which to do some controlled, prospective studies. Animal models represent one approach to this problem. In these systems some of the potentially important variables can be isolated and studied both individually and in relationship to each other.

Another clinical consideration relevant to animal modeling research is that the defining characteristics of depression are largely phenomenological. That is, even though it is an affective illness, there are measurable behavioral and social changes that can serve as indices.

Given the multiplicity of conceptual models and of variables, no single animal model of depression is going to be sufficient. Depression is a multivariate illness, and the term itself is heterogenous. The syndrome includes a large number of signs, symptoms, affects, cognitive disturbances, social disturbances, and neurobiological abnormalities which no single experimental model can encompass. For example, a model that might permit brain mechanism studies may not permit social or developmental studies. Other socially based models may be more appropriate for certain kinds of mechanism studies than others. Advocates of one or another approach need to stop criticizing each other's work in destructive ways and recognize the advantages and limitations of the multiple models. This is especially true given the nature of the depressive syndromes. An attitude which unfortunately is becoming more prominent is to view major depressions as genetic–neurobiological illnesses and to evaluate models solely on the basis of their ability to facilitate research in these areas. While one should not underrate the considerable research advances in these areas, depressions, even major ones, occur in a social context, and social–developmental models are also needed.

There are some specific clinical research issues in which animal models can help, and these should be kept in mind when reading the subsequent discussion of specific models. The following discussion is certainly not comprehensive but represents some specialized, clinical considerations to take into account when considering approaches to modeling human depression in animals.

The first issue concerns the influence of developmental events on the emergence of depressions later in life. Historically, this area has focused on the role of early loss or separations in humans as sensitizing events. This literature has been reviewed elsewhere (Akiskal and McKinney, 1975; Paykel, 1982) and is complex and controversial. There are significant methodological debates and, unfortunately, the lines tend to get drawn between those with a more neurobiological orientation and those with a more psychosocial or psychodynamic view of affective disorders. At the risk of doing an injustice to such a volatile area, the following general conclusions can be drawn: (a) There are now data from well-controlled studies that show that "exit-type life events" in general precede nonbipolar depressions at greater than control rates. (b) Interpersonal loss, or separation, while certainly not specific to depressions, does have a special relationship with nonbipolar depressions (i.e., is a risk factor). (c) The presence or absence of life events (e.g., separation) is independent of the symptom pattern. That is, the depression with an endogenous symptom pattern is just as likely or unlikely to have been preceded by a loss. Another way to say this is that the understanding of a life event such as separation or object loss is just as important for endogenous depressions as for so-called reactive ones. (d) The presence, or absence, of a life event such as separation bears very little relationship to treatment response to medication. Numerous studies show that response to antidepressant medication is largely predicted by symptom pattern (or other variables such as family history), which in turn is independent of life events. For example, a person with a clear object loss, but with an endogenous symptom pattern, would be as likely to respond to medication as a person with an endogenous symptom pattern but no precipitant. Animal models have led to the accumulation of data about this question, and these studies are reviewed in the section on separation. Thus, one clinical rationale for separation studies in primates comes from the probable importance of separation as a risk factor for several kinds of human depression, maybe especially childhood depressions. Using animal paradigms it is now possible to evaluate some of the variables—developmental, social, and neurobiological—influencing the response to separation. Most of these kinds of studies cannot be done in humans, and therefore it has been difficult to evaluate the influencing variables in a prospective design. Quite apart from any possible linkage between depression and separation, the separation paradigm in animals represents an additional way to evaluate the effects of a powerful social stressor on a specified set of behaviors and on neurobiological functioning. This reasoning properly takes the work out of irresolvable debates about the validity of the separation model as a model for human depression. There is no such thing as a model for depression or, for that matter, for any form of psychopathology. Rather, there is a need to redirect our thinking to the development and study of limited animal preparations for studying certain specific aspects of human psychopathology in ways that cannot be done in humans. This is the proper clinical framework in which to view separation studies. A somewhat newer clinical research issue concerns the role of developmental object loss as an etiological factor in the group of chronic depressives. Akiskal (Rosenthal and Akiskal, 1981; Akiskal *et al.*, 1978) has pioneered in the development of this concept, and animal models could be developed for additional evaluation of this theory, especially regarding how such events interact with neurobiological functioning.

Another important clinical research issue concerns the influence of social or interpersonal events as etiological factors in depression. Recent research has strongly suggested an important role for a number of such factors (Brown *et al.*, 1973a, 1973b, 1979; Paykel, 1974, 1978, 1979a, 1979b, 1982), but the research is controversial and frequently discounted by those with neurobiological orientations. This is unfortunate since animal preparations are now available for evaluating some of these factors and how they relate to neurobiological functioning.

An additional clinical consideration involves the study of the cognitive aspects of depression (Beck, 1967). Beck's theory postulates that feelings of helplessness and hopelessness are core features of clinical depressions. Rather than being secondary manifestations of a disordered emotional state—depression—the emotional state of depression is secondary to the altered cognitions. According to this theory, the thinking patterns of the depressive are characterized by a "cognitive triad" consisting of a negative conception of the self, negative interpretations of one's experiences, and a negative view of the future. Increasingly, the role of such factors, whether they are one's view of oneself as helpless and hopeless or actual cognitive deficits, are recognized as central phenomena. The learned helplessness models in animals relate closely to these theories, although there is a need to develop other models to evaluate possible learning deficits in this context.

Another important clinical consideration relates to the neurotransmitter theories of depression (Bunney and Davis, 1965; Coppen, 1968; Coppen and Shaw, 1963; Coppen et al., 1966; Janowsky et al., 1972; Lapin and Oxenkrug, 1969; Prange, 1964; Schildkraut, 1965; Whybrow and Mendels, 1969). We have gone from a single deterministic view of neurotransmitters in relationship to depression to a proliferation of complex theories involving multiple systems and their interaction. It is still not known which possible changes are trait related and which are state related. That is, to what extent do certain neurotransmitter alterations serve as markers or predictors of depression, and to what extent are they state-related markers reflecting the state of depression, no matter how produced. Also, there are no data from humans regarding the influence of neurotransmitters on a variety of responses to social stressors. These are complicated interrelationships but are reasonable topics for investigation in appropriate experimental systems in animals.

Perhaps the most important clinical consideration in the development of animal models of depression involves theory building. Our ability to accumulate data has far outstripped our ability to conceptualize and to develop theories to explain the data. By systematically studying one variable at a time while controlling others, and then studying variables in combination, it should become possible to develop more reasonable theories of the affective disorders than we have at present. We have all paid insufficient attention to theory building despite the existence of a significant literature on this topic (Dubin, 1969).

Pharmacological Models of Depression

One of the oldest, and still most widely used, approaches to developing animal models of human depressions involves the administration of drugs to animals in order to reproduce some of the symptoms of human depression. A related approach uses drugs to produce a set of changes in animals that do not necessarily bear much phenomenological similarity to human depressions. This approach nevertheless has high empirical validity in terms of predicting clinical drug responses. Porsolt (1982), in reviewing this area, speaks of yet a third class of animal models. This heterogenous class, while not based on drug-induced changes, has been useful for predicting and characterizing antidepressant activity. These models have high empirical validity in terms of drug screening but, in terms of induction techniques or behaviors, seemingly bear little relationship to depression. Porsolt mentions such examples as muricide behavior, the bulbectomized rat syndrome, and kindled amygdaloid convulsions as belonging in this category. Table 1 illustrates some of the pharmacologically induced animal models of depression.

As far as drug induction models go, the syndrome induced by reserpine and related compounds has been the most widely used. Reserpine, when given to various animal species, produces a characteristic set of behaviors including ptosis, hypothermia, huddling, inactivity, social withdrawal, and sedation. These, and other behavioral changes, have been likened to human depression. The other historical context for the interest in this model came from the clinical observation that reserpine-containing drugs could induce depression in humans taking them for the treatment of hypertension (Freis, 1954; Limieux, Davignon, and Genst, 1956). This observation, at least in its initial form, has been called into question on the basis of later evidence (Goodwin and Bunney,

Table 1 Pharmacologically Induced Animal Models of Depression

	Behaviors	Drug-response issues
Reserpine	Ptosis Hypothermia Inactivity	Central vs peripheral effects
	Social withdrawal Sedation	Historical screen
Amphetamine (withdrawal)	Motor activity Self-stimulation behavior	Reversed by ami, imi, mianserin, pargyline Better reversal with chronic administration
Clonidine	Hypothermia Analgesia Sedation	
	Hypoactivity	Antidepressant screen?
Amine-potentiation	Not involved	Mainly physiological

1971). It appears that the humans who get depressed while taking reserpine-containing drugs are those who have a previous history of depressions and presumably a vulnerability in this area.

Porsolt (1982) and others (Colpaert, Lenaerts, Niemegeers, and Janssen, 1975; Garattini and Jori, 1967; Howard, Soroko, and Cooper, 1981) have provided extensive reviews of the reserpine syndrome as an animal model of depression. In addition, a number of related compounds have been used to induce symptoms qualitatively similar to those produced by reserpine although a number of factors differ—the speed of onset, the duration, central versus peripheral effects, etc. The arguments about the validity of the reserpine model have been based largely on the effects of psychotropic drugs on the behaviors induced by administration of reserpine and related drugs. Thus, the validity questions regarding this model center about its empirical validity.

There is an extensive literature about the antagonism of reserpine-induced activity (Porsolt, 1982). Initially, it was thought that most clinically active antidepressant drugs antagonized some or all of the symptoms induced by reserpine and thus that the model had high empirical validity. In general, this still remains true, but there are a number of inconsistencies that limit general conclusions. As a matter of fact, the reserpine syndrome itself is not a unitary entity. There are many different effects involved. For example, ptosis antagonism, although probably a peripheral effect, seems to detect the greatest number of clinically effective antidepressants, including some of the newer antidepressants that appear to be false negatives in other reserpine procedures. In evaluating the empirical validity of the reserpine model we must therefore be specific about which behaviors are involved. Some behaviors might have high validity in terms of predicting clinical drug response, but the mediating mechanisms might not be central in origin. This particular animal preparation would therefore not lend itself well to central mechanism studies but might be useful for screening large numbers of drugs. Reserpine has so many different neurochemical effects that it is difficult to determine which mechanism is associated with which behaviors.

There are several other pharmacologically induced models which have been proposed. One is the amphetamine withdrawal model (Kokkinidis, Zacharko, and Predy, 1980; Lynch and Leonard, 1978; Seltzer and Tongre, 1975). Animals which have been subjected to repeated amphetamine treatments show decreases in motor activity and in self-stimulation behavior when the drug is stopped. These effects can be reversed by amitriptyline, imipramine, mianserin, and pargyline to a certain extent when given on an acute basis but especially when given on a chronic basis.

Clonidine-induced behavioral depression is being explored as another pharmacological model (Delini-Stula *et al.*, 1979; Gower and Marriott, 1980; Green *et al.*, 1982; Hunt *et al.*, 1981; Robson, *et al.*, 1978; Von Voigtlander *et al.*, 1978). Clonidine, an alpha-adrenergic receptor stimulant, is thought to act at presynaptic receptor sites to inhibit the release of norepinephrine. This results in hypothermia, analgesia, and marked sedation. The hypoactivity following clonidine administration in particular has been proposed as a test model for antidepressant drugs. There are some conflicting results about which class of drugs are effective in this model, but, in a spectrum of pharmacologically induced models, it may play a role in screening some antidepressants that might be inactive in other models.

An additional class of pharmacological induction procedures involves the potentiation, by antidepressants, of the behavioral and other effects of amines or their precursors (Moller-Nielsen, 1980; Sanghvi and Gershon, 1977). These procedures do not even attempt to mimic the clinical condition but are based on existing theories about the role of these amines in the etiology of depression. Thus, they are mainly theory-driven procedures to learn more about how amines interact with each other and how they are influenced by antidepressant drugs. By such routes important information may be obtained that may ultimately bear on mechanism questions and that can even be tested later in more highly developed behavioral models. Examples of such procedures include the potentiation by antidepressants of the various central effects of amphetamine and of yohimbine. New tests in this area are being developed almost constantly, and this book cannot review them in any detail except to point out the basic strategy involved and how it relates to a spectrum of approaches to animal modeling.

There are a number of other empirically based pharmacological models that have not been proposed as resembling depression but which are being evaluated strictly for their empirical validity. The number of such tests has multiplied recently, in part, as a result of the failure of more classical tests to detect antidepressant activity of some newer classes of antidepressants. Examples include muricide behavior in rats (Sanghvi, 1977; Vogel, 1975), the bulbectomized rat syndrome (Cairncross *et al.*, 1978; Van Riezen, Schnieden, and Wren, 1977;), kindled amygdaloid convulsions (Babington, 1977; Stach, Lazarova, and Kacz, 1980), and REM sleep preparations in cats (Scherschlicht *et al.*, 1982). Undoubtedly more will be developed in the search for newer classes of antidepressant drugs and as our understanding of the neurobiology of depression broadens.

In summary, pharmacologically induced models have been, and

continue to be, important for screening clinically effective drugs. Thus, they should be evaluated for their empirical or predictive validity. None is perfect since each has a certain proportion of false negatives and false positives, but by using a battery of such tests an even higher degree of empirical validity may be achieved.

In the case of all empirically based tests we should keep in mind that we cannot necessarily reason from the mechanism by which the drug presumably acts in the animal preparation to its mechanism of action in human depression. There are potentially too many intervening variables, and additional types of animal preparations may be necessary to assist with mechanism questions.

Separation Models

It is likely that humans and many animal species are in their most stable condition when they have developed secure social attachment systems. Disruption of these attachment systems has by now been established as a very stressful event which almost invariably leads to the development of grief reactions and, in some vulnerable individuals, can serve as a risk factor for the development of clinical depressions. The reaction to separation is influenced by, among others, developmental, social, and neurobiological variables. Sorting out the influence of these variables, and how they might interact with each other, has been extremely difficult to do in humans. Investigators have therefore turned to animal models for a more systematic study of the behavioral and, more recently, neurobiological effects of separation.

The earliest work on separation in animals began in the 1960s. Jensen and Tolman (1962) reported the effects of separating pigtail macaque (*M. nemestrina*) infants from their mothers at the ages of 5 and 7 months for short periods and then reuniting them with their own or another mother. Other laboratories also did separation studies in the 1960s. For example, Seay, Hansen, and Harlow (1962) reported the effects of separating infant rhesus monkeys (M. mulatta) from their mothers for longer periods. In both of the above cases the separations were highly traumatic for the infants. The behaviors were divided into two categories labeled "protest" and "despair." The protest stage, which occurred immediately after the separation, was characterized by such changes as marked increases in vocalization and locomotion, and by attempts to return to the mother if she was visible. Monkeys were often so agitated during this stage that they would not eat or drink properly.

This stage typically lasted 24–48 hours and was followed by the despair, or "depression," stage. During this phase the monkeys showed significant decreases on locomotion and vocalization. They became socially withdrawn and showed increases in a variety of self-directed behaviors such as huddling. Food and water intake could drop to dangerous levels during this phase, and animals would often die if electrolyte and nutritional balance was not properly maintained. The protest and despair responses in rhesus monkeys following maternal separation has been likened to the responses in human children as described by Spitz (1946), Bowlby (1961, 1960a, 1960b), the Robertsons (1971), and Robertson and Bowlby (1952), who observed children in institutions (usually hospitals or nurseries) where they were unavoidably separated from their parents and families. Spitz applied the term *anaclitic* depression to these children (Spitz, 1946). The stages of response to separation were described by the Robertsons as protest, despair, and denial (later changed to detachment). Bowlby incorporated these stages into his theory of primary separation anxiety, with the reaction to separation being conceptualized in terms of attachment system theory, which was being developed at that time, although up to this time there was no suggestion of separation as a model for certain aspects of human depression.

About this same time Kaufman and Rosenblum (1967a, 1967b, 1968) began their pioneering studies of the separation reactions of bonnet and pigtail macaques. Their technique of studying separation was different from that just described. In the previous studies mothers and infants had typically been housed in dyadic pairs and the separation accomplished by removing the infant to another cage. In the Kaufman–Rosenblum paradigm, mothers and infants lived as a group, and separation was generally accomplished by mother removal, leaving the infant behind in its usual social group but without its biological mother.

When the infants were 5 to 6 months of age, the mothers were removed from the pen where the animals had been reared as a group since birth. The separations took place at different times, with some overlap of separations between subjects. The authors reported a clear "agitation" phase as well as a subsequent "depression" phase which were roughly similar to the stages reported by Seay, Hansen, and Harlow. Agitation was marked by distress vocalizations, high levels of locomotion, and increased digit sucking. Depression consisted of decreases in activity, increases in huddled nonlocomotive behavior and a general state of social withdrawal. The above reaction was typical for pigtail macaque infants but not for bonnet infants. Bonnet infants had a much less severe response to separation in that they did not show evidence of the despair stage as did the pigtail infants. This was interpreted as being due to the differences in their species-specific social and bonding behavior. The pigtail infants formed strong dyadic bonds, whereas the bonnets had more substitute caretaking and group mothering. When a bonnet's mother was removed, the infant would form attachments with other adult females. That was not a natural behavior for the pigtail infants, and they showed the depressive behaviors. More recent work has shown that depressive behavior in the bonnet infant can be induced if there is cross-species rearing and no substitute caretaking available.

Hinde and colleagues (1966) played a major role in developing the mother–infant separation paradigm in primates. Their findings were roughly similar to those described above. They initially reported the effects of removal for 6 days of the mothers of four, 8-month-old infants from stable pen-housed groups of one adult male and four or five adult female rhesus monkeys. They noted that the separation was accompanied by increases in vocalizations and a transient increase in locomotion. After the first day, locomotion scores dropped precipitously to below preseparation levels, along with decreased levels of social interaction and environmental manipulation. The authors suggested that their data, while showing no detachment response, agreed with Bowlby's formulation of protest and despair responses to maternal separation. This same group also studied the effects of mother removal for 6 days in 19 rhesus monkey infants at the ages of 18, 21, 25, and 30 weeks. During the separation, infants of all ages showed decreased locomotor activity, suppression of play, and decreased environmental manipulation. The authors noted two caveats, however. First, they found a high degree of individual variability in the behavior of infants, and, second, they cautioned against projecting the meaning of their data onto studies of longer-term separations. Both of these caveats, especially the one regarding individual variability, are well taken in view of recent research. The issue of individual variability has proven to be one of the most meaningful to investigate in primate separation studies, and this is where some of the most significant links to our understanding of human separations are being made. At an earlier stage in the separation research literature, the issue of individual variability, viewed as troublesome, was not examined in any intensive way. It is now known that there is significant individual variability in the response to attachment bond disruption in animals, just as there is in humans, and rather than ignore it, the sources of this multiple variability are important to understand from developmental and neurobiological frameworks.

Hinde and colleagues (1970, 1972, 1974), in addition to reporting the existence of protest and despair stages, reported that preseparation behavior helped to predict behavior after separation and that sex of the infants may also influence the response to maternal separation, with male infants responding more severely than females. In these studies, rhesus mothers were removed from their infants, which were left in the same social group, for either 6 or 13 days when the infants were 20–32 weeks old. After the mother's removal, the infants exhibited high levels of distress calling. This distress calling was extremely high on the day of the mother's removal and decreased somewhat over the rest of the separation period but, in the case of all infants, was still higher a month after the mother's return than it had been during the preseparation period. During the separation phase, the infants also showed a reduction in locomotor activity and a characteristic hunched posture resembling huddling in some other studies. When the mother was returned, the infant would try to cling to and spend more time on the mother than before. The mother would initially allow some of this and then reject the infant for a while before the two would gradually come to some sort of mutually acceptable readjustment. There was marked individual variability in the extent to which long-term disturbances in the mother–infant relationship persisted.

When the period of separation was 13 days, rather than 6, the effect on the infant was more severe and long lasting. However, the issue of individual variability was commented on as an important one in these studies. One source of this variability in the response to separation from the biological mother was thought to be the prior nature of the mother–infant relationship. Hinde developed what he called a "distress index" and related this index to preseparation measures of mother–infant interaction. The measures that went into the distress index included the frequency of distress calls, locomotor activity, and the time spent in the hunched, depressive posture.

The key findings from this work were as follows:

1. The distress index was highly correlated between the different phases of the experiment. That is, the infants who ranked highest on these measures during the preseparation period also ranked highest during the separation phase. However, the separation experience increased the distress index in these infants, so one interpretation of these data was that the separation experience was acting to exacerbate tendencies present before the separation.
2. There were significant correlations between the distress index and the relative frequency of rejections and the infant's role in maintaining proximity. This has been referred to as "tension" in the mother–infant relationship. The separation data indicated

that the distress index was greatest in those infants which had the most "tense" relationship with their mothers. The infants which were most distressed during separation were those that were rejected most and had to play the greatest role in maintaining proximity to their mothers. There was also a high correlation between the distress index and measures of current mother–infant relationship after return of the mother to the infant. In other words, the distress index after separation was related to both preseparation measures of the mother–infant relationship as well as to contemporaneous measures of the mother–infant relationship. The distress index immediately after reunion was more closely related to the preseparation measures, and little to contemporaneous ones. As Hinde points out, however, with the passage of time the relationship of the distress index with contemperaneous measures became stronger, and that with preseparation measures weaker.

3. This same group has also found that short-term maternal separation, early in development, has long-term effects some 2 to 3 years later, even without any intervening separations. This study involved comparing control infants with no history of maternal separation with infants which had had one or two 6-day separations when they were 30–32 weeks old. Subsequent comparisons were made when the infants were 12 or 30 months old, that is, 6 months or 2 years after the separation experience. The mother–infant relationship at 12 months did not differ between the two groups, with the exception that the previously separated animals showed less locomotor activity. In the home cage, the two groups did not differ in their readiness to approach strange objects, but in a strange indoor cage the previously separated infants were significantly less ready to approach strange objects. Animals with a history of two 6-day separations differed from nonseparated controls more than those with only one separation. At 30 months, similar differences were found. Thus, a separation experience of only 6 days, and especially two such separation experiences, can affect behavior 6 months and even 2 years later. However, it requires a challenge for the effects to become manifest. Baseline behaviors do not differ much from controls with no history of separation. This interesting finding is consistent with a developing line of clinical theory regarding the possible sensitizing role of a variety of aversive early experiences. The effects are long term in nature but only manifest themselves under challenge conditions.

As primate researchers extended their original work on the response to maternal separation, it became apparent that the response of monkey infants was influenced by a number of parameters. As previously mentioned, work with bonnet macaques indicated that species of the infant is an important variable.

Age and social conditions also affect the response to maternal separation. When rhesus infants were separated from their mothers at 60, 90, and 120 days of age, all subjects showed a typical protest and despair response, but the infants which had been separated at 90 days showed a much more severe response than those that had been separated at other ages (Suomi, Collins, and Harlow, 1973). In addition, infants housed in single-cage units during the separation period showed a much more severe behavioral response to separation than infants housed with a peer. Follow-up observations indicated that these differences lasted to, and even worsened by, 6 months of age (Suomi, 1976; Suomi, Collins, Harlow, and Ruppenthal, 1976).

Kaplan (1970) separated squirrel monkeys from their mothers at 13–22 weeks of age, a time when physical contact between the mother and infant is at a low level. In this study, mother–infant pairs had been housed in individual cages rather than as a group. The separation had only transient effects on the behavior of either mother or infant. The infants had an initial period of excitement following separation that seemed to resemble the protest stage in macaques. However, after this initial period the behavior of both mother and infants returned to preseparation levels with no evidence of the despair stage. It is unclear whether these differences in the reaction to separation in squirrel monkeys are because of species differences, differences in age, or perhaps other variables. It is increasingly clear that even within a given species, individual variability is a major issue, and additional studies directed at understanding the sources for this variability are needed.

Neurobiological Effects of Maternal Separation

The reaction to maternal separation is a biobehavioral syndrome involving not only behavioral effects but also major neurobiological changes.

Reite and associates (Reite, 1977; Reite, Kaufman, Pauley and Stynes, 1974; Reite, Seiler, Crowley, Hydinger-MacDonald, and Short, 1982; Reite, Short, Seiler, and Pauley, 1981) have done a series of studies of pigtail macaque infants undergoing maternal separation. Using totally implanted multichannel biotelemetry systems, they have studied heart rate, body temperature, and sleep physiology of the infants before, during, and after separation from their mothers. Separation is generally accomplished by removing the biological mother from a group living situation and leaving the infant in the group. From a behavioral standpoint, they, like others, have found that attachment bonds are as central to the development of monkeys as they are to people. Experimental disruption of these bonds leads to serious changes. For example, there were significant increases in the infant's heart rate and body temperature immediately after maternal separation (Reite, Short, Kaufman, Stynes, and Pauley, 1978). These changes were most pronounced early in separation and tended to diminish as the separation continued. Beginning with the first night, both the heart rate and body temperature decreased from baseline levels and the behavioral patterns became more depressive. During reunion both the heart rate and body temperature returned to normal, although some infants had lower heart rates well into the reunion. This research group has also reported an increased incidence of cardiac arrythmias resulting from separation. Significant sleep changes have also been reported to occur during maternal separation, including increased sleep latency, more frequent arousals, less total sleep, and a disruption of REM sleep. (Reite and Short, 1977, 1978; Reite, Stynes, Vaughn, Pauley, and Short, 1976).

Other research has examined some neurochemical effects in rhesus monkey infants in the protest stage following maternal separation (Breese, Smith, Mueller, Howard, Prange, Lipton, Young, McKinney, and Lewis, 1973). While infant rhesus monkeys were showing most of the classic behavioral signs of the protest stage, they were sacrificed and regional brain dissections done. The adrenal glands were also examined for levels of catecholamine-synthesizing enzymes. Significant findings included elevated serotonin levels in the hypothalamus plus significantly higher levels in the adrenal gland of all of the major enzymes involved in catecholamine synthesis. Resting levels of norepinephrine and dopamine were unchanged in any of the brain regions examined. This study measured resting levels of these substances at one point in time and thus gives no information about possible dynamic changes occuring over time. However, it provides additional confirmation of the powerful effects of maternal attachment bond disruption. The syndrome is neither transient, mild, superficial, nor limited to one aspect part of the animals physiology.

The effects of maternal separation on the corticoid response have been examined in squirrel monkeys (Coe, Mendoza, Smotherman, and

Levine, 1978; Levine, Coe, and Smotherman, 1978; Smotherman, Hunt, McGinnis, and Levine, 1979; Vogt and Levine, 1980). Brief separations (30 minutes) from the mother, or from a surrogate, produced a marked increase in the pituitary–adrenal response. Initially, identical physiological responses were found whether the infant was separated from a mother or a surrogate. The real mother also showed an elevated corticoid response to separation. This latter finding is interesting in that the mothers' responses to infant removal has been minimally described in most studies. The attention has been on the infant. Typically the mother has been described as acutely upset but returning to normal very quickly. The infants corticoid response was thought to be due to the separation itself rather than the new cage in which it was housed during the separation phase, although, as seen later, caging arrangements can affect the behavioral and hormonal responses to separation. It also appears that infants of the highly dominant mothers were the ones that showed the greatest adrenocortical response to separation. In a later report concerning separation distress in surrogate-reared squirrel monkeys, it was found that separation from the surrogate resulted in a behavioral response but no cortisol response, whereas separation from the real mother resulted in both a behavioral and a cortisol response.

Depending on the specifics of how the study is done, the behavioral and hormonal responses to the stress of maternal separation can vary. For example, if a squirrel monkey infant is housed proximally to its mother, it will have very high levels of distress calling but not nearly as much adrenal activation as when the separation is combined with isolation from the mother. The latter condition results in considerable adrenal activation but far less distress calling. These investigators make the important point that if one was relying solely on distress vocalizations, one might be mislead regarding the nature of the stress being experienced. They have also found that the acute response, as reflected in adrenal activation, to maternal separation in squirrel monkeys is diminished by social companionship in the home environment.

This same research group has found that treatment with dexamethasone, which blocks adrenocorticotropic hormone (ACTH) output and thereby lowers cortisol output, results in a significant reduction in the vocal response following separation.

There are also some data from this group (Coe, Wiener, Rosenberg, and Levine, 1985) as well as from Reite and colleagues that separation affects the immune system. Reite, Harbeck, and Hoffman (1981) had previously found that an 11-day separation could affect immune function in macaques, as measured by the proliferative response of lymphocytes to mitogen stimulation. Coe *et al.* (1985) found that in both housing conditions (i.e., housed alone in an unfamiliar environment within sight of other separated infants vs housed as a group in the home cage after removal of the mothers), separation resulted in a decrease in C3 and C4 (complement protein) levels by 7 days after maternal loss. However, the decrease in the individually housed monkeys was significantly greater, lasted longer, and was more consistently found. Separation also resulted in a significant decrease in serum levels of immunoglobins, although there was no differential housing condition effect. It also appears, on the basis of data available so far, that separation stress has a strong effect on antibody production, as assessed by an antigen challenge using a benign bacteriophage which evokes a reliable T-dependent response.

This important research illustrates the complexity of the relationship between neurobiological and behavioral changes accompanying separation. They may not always change together under the same conditions, and we cannot necessarily rely on one index alone. In addition, it is important to obtain adequate baseline behavioral profiles of both the group structure and individuals.

Further evidence that mother–infant separation in macaques is a useful experimental model of depression comes from studies with *Macaca fasicularis*. It has been shown that desipramine is effective in preventing the typical protest and despair behaviors in separated infants in this species (Hrdina *et al.*, 1979).

When infant langur monkeys (*Presbytis entellus*) were separated from their mothers at 6–8 months of age, all infants showed changes in social behavior. The reactions varied from minimal to severe and included two deaths. All infants sought out substitute caretaking during the separation and adopted a major substitute caretaker. Most infants actually remained with the substitute even when the original caretaker returned. (Dolhinow, 1980).

Important work relevant to understanding maternal separation has been done in a number of other species. Hofer and Ackerman, in a series of studies of separation of rat pups, found major psychophysiological changes as part of the response to maternal separation (Ackerman, Hofer, and Weiner, 1979; Hofer, 1970, 1975a, 1975b, 1975c, 1976). Cardiac and respiratory rates decreased about 40% during the first 12–16 hours after 2-week-old rat pups were separated from their mothers. Body weight and temperature also declined for 3 days in all separated animals. These researchers also studied sleep changes and found an increase in time spent awake, reduction of REM sleep, and increased frequency of state transitions with shorter and more frequent periods of both slow-wave sleep and REM sleep. If the rat pups survived, on reunion all of these measures returned to those characteristic of normally mothered infants. Of special interest in this work is the concept that the sensory processes underlying attachment and their disruption may be important in understanding separation responses.

Additional maternal separation studies have been done using canine puppies, guinea pigs, and chicks (Panksepp, Herman, Conner, Bishop, and Scott, 1978; Panksepp, Vilberg, Bean, Coy, and Kastin, 1978; Pettijohn, 1979; Pettijohn, Wong, Ebert, and Scott, 1977). From this work has developed a theory that brain endorphins may play a critical role in the mediation of social bonds and that when these bonds are disrupted by separation, a syndrome much like that following narcotics withdrawal is produced. In this work, distress vocalizations were used as an index of separation distress, and the effects of many pharmacological agents on these vocalizations were studied. In general, the distress vocalizations are reported to be relieved by morphine and made worse by the narcotic antagonist naloxone. A variety of opiate-like peptides have been tested, and all were effective, like morphine, in decreasing distress vocalizations in separated animals when injected in quite low doses into the vicinity of the fourth ventricle. The drugs were divided into the following three categories: (a) those which had no effect in reducing distress vocalizations—pentobarbital, imipramine; (b) those which decreased distress vocalizations—morphine, pilocarpine, quipazine, clonidine, chlordiazepoxide. Haloperidol, chlorpromazine, and apomorphine had small effects in terms of decreasing distress vocalizations; (c) those which increased distress vocalizations—naloxone, atropine, and methysergide. The opiate system was found to have the most powerful effect on distress vocalization of all the systems studied.

Peer Separation Studies

Another approach to separation studies developed in recent years is the peer separation model. Rhesus monkeys, and most other primate species, develop strong and complex social bonds, and paradigms have been developed that involve experimental disruption of these bonds in peers of various ages, including adults (Bowden and McKinney, 1972; McKinney, Suomi, and Harlow, 1972; Mineka and Suomi, 1978; Suomi, Eisele, Grady, and Harlow, 1975; Suomi, Harlow, and Domek, 1970). In general, the behavioral reaction to peer separation is quite similar to that of maternal separation in terms of the classic protest–despair response. Furthermore, when peer groups are formed and repetitive separations done, the response is obtainable with each separation. Not surprisingly, a number of variables can influence the nature of the response. These include age, rearing conditions, housing conditions before, during, and after each separation, and treatment with pharmacological agents. As background for the next section, which focuses on a summary of the relevance of the separation models to human depression, the basic findings from peer separation studies are summarized.

From a behavioral standpoint, monkeys respond initially to peer separation with a period of hyperactivity. Locomotion and vocalization scores increase significantly, and the animals can appear quite agitated. This lasts 24–36 hours and is followed by a period when the animals huddle, are socially withdrawn, activity drops, and food and water intake decline to levels that can be dangerous. There is an increase in self-directed behaviors and a decreased responsiveness to the external environment. A number of variables can influence the response to peer separation, and these have been reviewed by Mineka and Suomi (1978). Thus far, peer separation has been studied mostly in rhesus monkeys, so species differences cannot be assessed. Age does not appear to be an important variable within the first year of life, although some reports suggest that the separation response is worse when it is done at about 90 days of age. Sex differences have not been systematically evaluated. Peer separations can be done repeatedly without any worsening or lessening of the effect across a large number of separations.

Developmental variables are important. Two separate studies (Suomi, 1976; Kraemer, 1985) have found that peer-reared monkeys responded to peer separations more severely than monkeys which were reared with their mothers for the first several months of life and then put into peer groups.

Some of the individual variability can also be related to neurobiological variables. For example, cerebrospinal fluid norepinephrine (CSF NE) appears to be a trait-related marker predicting a more severe response to separations. Animals with lower CSF NE levels respond to separation with more huddling and self-directed behaviors than animals with higher levels. By contrast CSF homovanillic acid and CSF 5-hydroxyindoleacetic acid are state-related markers which reflect the behavioral response to peer separation.

Pharmacological agents can also affect the response to peer separation. Table 2 summarizes the influence of pharmacological agents on the response to peer separation as well as that of opiate-like peptides on the maternal separation responses discussed previously.

Imipramine will reverse the reaction to peer separation and prevent the reaction to future separations as long as the monkeys are kept on it (Suomi, Seaman, Lewis, Delizio, and McKinney, 1978). They return to more typical separation behavior when it is withdrawn.

Amphetamine modifies the behavioral response to separation in a

Table 2 Influence of Pharmacological Agents
on Separation Response[a]

	Protest	Despair
Imipramine	Decreases	Decreases
AMPT	?	Increases
PCPA	No effect	No effect
Fusaric acid	?	Decreases
Amphetamine	?	Decreases
Alcohol	?	Decreases (low dose) Increases (high dose)
Opiate-like peptides	Decreases	?
Naloxone	Increases	?

[a]AMPT—alpha-methyl-paratyrosine; PCPA—para-chlorophenylalanine.

very similar manner to imipramine, but the overall effects of the two
drugs on group social behavior can be distinguished. The dose level of
amphetamine that is effective in altering the separation response is also
very disruptive to ongoing social behavior in the group situation. This is
not true for imipramine. Alpha-methyl-paratyrosine (AMPT), which
lowers norepinephrine and dopamine levels, makes the separation response much more severe, and it does so at doses that have no effect in
the group-housing situation or in chronically singly caged animals
which are not undergoing the stress of separations. Para-chlorophenylalanine (PCPA), which blocks serotonin synthesis, has no effect
(Kraemer and McKinney, 1979).

Low doses of alcohol alleviate the peer separation response, whereas high doses make it worse (Kraemer and McKinney, 1981).

There are still many aspects of the peer separation response that are
unexplored. For example, Maxim (1980) reared pigtail macaques in pairs
rather than in a group. At 4 weeks of age electrodes were placed in the
anterolateral hypothalamus positive reward site. Peer separations were
done at 4 months of age. The behavioral syndrome produced, much like
that in the Kaplan (1970) and in the Lewis *et al.* (1976) studies, was
nonphasic and more like "agitation–tension–fear." Stimulation at the
reward site known to reduce these fear behaviors did indeed significntly
decrease such behaviors exhibited by the separated animals in this
study, and the infants bar pressed more frequently to obtain such
stimulation.

Much of the same work which has been done with the maternal separation model needs to be done with the peer separation model; however, the data available so far suggest the peer separation model as a reasonable approach for studying the effects of attachment bond disruption in an experimental system in animals. As seen in the next section, such paradigms have potential clinical significance, although their more fundamental importance is as a paradigm for investigating the behavioral and neurobiological effects of a specified behavioral event.

Several theoretical conceptualizations of separation phenomena have been offered. However, space permits only a brief summary of the theories. They can be organized into four categories as follows (after Mineka and Suomi, 1978): (a) attachment-object loss theory, (b) conservation–withdrawal theory, (c) learned helplessness theory, and (d) opponent-process theory. Reviews of these theories are included in the list of references at the end of this chapter.

1. *The attachment-object loss approach to separation.* Bowlby's theories about separation derive from his earlier writings about attachment behavior. Basically, he argues that one of the chief functions of an attachment object is that of providing a base of security; when the attachment object is no longer there, the base of security is gone. This is a very unpleasant experience and, according to Bowlby, results in a universal separation response. The response is one of distress or protest followed by despair, when the separation becomes extended. In general, Bowlby's theories provide an interesting theoretical framework within which to understand some of the primate separation literature. Indeed, parts of Bowlby's theories are based on the primate attachment–separation literature.

2. *The conservation–withdrawal theory.* This approach to understanding the primate separation literature says that faced with a stressful situation, such as separation, an organism first engages in a fight–flight reaction, and that the protest stage is best understood in this context. This response is adaptive in the sense that the agitation-type behaviors characteristic of this stage increase the likelihood of reunion because they draw attention to the infant or peer. However, this phase cannot last indefinitely and there then occurs an energy conservation stage (despair, depression) characterized by inactivity and withdrawal. This too is adaptive in the sense that it conserves resources and decreases the probability of detection by predators. In this framework, de-

spair is not the result of fatigue but occurs in order to prevent fatigue.

3. *The learned helplessness approach to separation.* It has been suggested that separation from an attachment object is one way of inducing a sense of helplessness because the attachment object is the major figure through which control over the environment is gained. There is a need for some direct studies in which the controllability of an organism's environment during separation is manipulated to further evaluate this theoretical explanation. However, this theory is an interesting attempt to bridge two levels of explanations of depression. The results of such studies will help in further understanding how cognitive–perceptual factors may serve as important mediators of the separation response.

4. *Opponent-process theory.* Solomon and Corbit have proposed that their opponent-process model of the temporal dynamics of affect and acquired motivation help to understand the changes that occur over time in the dynamics of attachment and separation behaviors. According to this theory, the changes seen following separation are a natural reaction typical of a normally functioning nervous system. The observed despair is analogous to the withdrawal symptoms shown by a heroin addict when he is separated from the drug. This theory says that when a nervous system is stimulated by any intense affect-arousing stimulus (e.g., exposure to an attachment object), there is a primary affective reaction (the "a" process) that has multiple components. Once this "a" process has been activated, a second process is automatically set into play to bring the organism back to hedonic neutrality (the "b" process). States are spoken of in relationship to the relative intensities of these processes. Specifically, as applied to attachment relationships, this theory says that prolonged or repeated exposure to an attachment object results in the strengthening of the "b" process. The theory goes on to say how separations cause State B to exist (State B only manifests itself when the "a" stimulus is gone and the "b" process is no longer opposed by the "a" process) and that State B is equated with despair. It is possible to develop predictions regarding the effects of repeated separations and of environmental variations, and these have been done. In general, they fit with the results of repeated separations of primates.

Separation Models: Rationale and Role in Modeling Studies

Table 3 summarizes the rationale for experimental studies of separation phenomena as well as their major behavioral and neurobiological effects. The initial rationale for doing separation studies had very little to do with their possible role as experimental systems in which to study certain aspects of human depression. Rather, they were a logical progression of a series of studies which demonstrated the importance of affectional or attachment systems in several animal species. Such systems are also important in humans irrespective of any controversies about depression, and herein lies the fundamental importance of animal separation studies. As mentioned before, having secure attachment systems is important for all species, including humans. In humans, such attachment systems inevitably get disrupted, and there are consequences. In animal systems, one can study the nature of such disruptions, and the various influences that can be brought to bear on them can be evaluated in a controlled way. In this context, the study of separation has fundamental importance for many areas of medicine that goes beyond any possible relationship with depression in particular.

Table 3 Experimental Studies of Separation

Rationale
  1. Study of a risk factor for human depressions
  2. Paradigm for study of stressful events
Behavioral effects
  Protest
    Increased activity
    Increased vocalizations
    Decreased food and water intake
  Despair
    Decreased activity
    Decreased vocalizations
    Increased social withdrawal
    Increased self-directed behaviors
    Decreased food and water intake
Neurobiological effects
  Increased plasma cortisol
  Increased adrenal catecholamine-synthesizing enzymes
  Increased hypothalamic serotonin
  Sleep disturbances
  Decreased body temperature
  Increased incidence of cardiac arrhythmias
  Decreased immune system function

Said another way, there are, in reality, two fundamental reasons to study separation phenomena. One is clinical and relates to the possibility that separation is one of the risk factors for human depressions. We do not have to assume any overall validity of the separation model to justify the study of it in this context.

In relation to depression models, the rationale for separation studies in animals thus derives from the evidence that strongly suggests social separations as risk factors that cut across types of depressions. The animal studies represent one way of examining these risk factors. There are obviously many other factors involved in depression; nevertheless, separations appear to be important events in vulnerable individuals and worthy of further study in some controlled experimental systems.

The second, and probably more important, reason is that the separation paradigm involves the use of a clear social induction of certain defined behaviors that can then be studied from developmental, social, and neurobiological frameworks.

In this context, separation studies may be prototypes for the study of stressful events in general and the role of stress factors in depressions. With the recent advances in our knowledge of the neurobiology of depression, it becomes increasingly important to have some experimental paradigms in which the interactions between neurobiological factors and social risk factors can be examined. This latter consideration is a cardinal reason for the continued study of separation models. In such animal preparations, there is the opportunity to control social and developmental variables and to do prospective studies of both behavioral and neurobiological parameters. The long-term effects of early alterations can be examined in a much shorter time. Repeated sampling of neurobiological measures (e.g., CSF) can be done in a manner not possible in humans and in relationship to specific units of behavior. One can also evaluate the effects of drugs on CSF parameters being studied in humans and what these changes mean in relation to specific social behaviors. There can also be clarification of the role of specific neurotransmitter systems in influencing specific units of social behavior including responses to separation. Humans are fundamentally social creatures, and an understanding of the social origins of psychopathology and how these origins are related to neurotransmitter systems becomes possible in this kind of preparation.

It should be noted that this conceptualization of separation studies does not make any *a priori* assumptions about their validity, on any level, in relation to human depression. Rather, it views them as experimental systems in which the relationship between a clear social inducer and subsequent behavioral and neurobiological changes can be examined.

As part of the development of the psychiatry of the future, it is critical to understand the ways in which behavior changes biochemistry and how the altered biochemistry in turn affects behavior. These are complex interrelationships, and our present language, conceptualization, and data leave a lot to be desired. However, studies designed to understand parts of these interrelationships need to be undertaken. Separation paradigms provide one way to do this.

To summarize, in a spectrum of approaches to animal modeling of depression, the major role of separation studies is to produce a given set of behaviors (many of which resemble the behaviors shown by human depressives) by way of a clearly defined induction technique (perhaps a major social risk factor). The neurobiological as well as behavioral effects of this experimental induction can be studied in ways that cannot be done in humans, and different intervention techniques can be tried and/or developed. Studies thus far point to similar profiles of pharmacological responsiveness as in human depressions. None of the above separation models, either singly or in aggregate, "proves" that these are valid models, but each in its own way provides a clear rationale for the continuing study of a fundamental human and animal phenomenon.

Uncontrollability Models

These particular models have been extensively studied for 15 or more years and relate closely to cognitive theories of human depression. Beck (1967) proposed a "cognitive triad" in depression, involving negative conception of the self, negative interpretations of one's experiences, and a negative view of the future. These are sometimes reflected in feelings of helplessness and hopelessness. Depressed patients often describe such feelings and thoughts. They feel that nothing they do matters and that they have no control over what happens to them. Whether these phenomena are primary or secondary is a moot question for the present discussion. The point is that they occur as core aspects of depression frequently enough to be worthy of additional experimental study. Etiological theories, as well as therapeutic approaches, have been suggested, based on this cognitive view of depression.

Actually, based on earlier work, it had been proposed that such a state of helplessness could be developed in animals. Richter (1957) reported that handling wild rats, which included clipping their whiskers and immersion in a swimming apparatus, induced sudden death. He speculated that such treatment resulted in the animals' being unable to either fight or flee—if you will, a state of "hopelessness."

This research area has become too large and complex to review in a comprehensive manner in this chapter. Uncontrollability models are sometimes known as "learned helplessness" models, though this term implies a mediating mechanism with which not all who work with uncontrollability models would agree.

In the original studies (Overmier and Seligman, 1967; Seligman and Maier, 1967) dogs were placed in one of three conditions. In the first condition, escapable shock, dogs were placed in harnesses and given electric shock. They were able to terminate the shock by touching a panel, and they learned to do so rather quickly. In the second condition, dogs were given inescapable shock. They were prepared as in the preceding condition, but when the shock was given they were unable to terminate it. Finally, in the third condition, dogs were placed in the harnesses but not shocked at all. This was a control for the effects of the shock itself. In phase two of the study, dogs were tested in a shuttle box and received shocks while unharnessed. Normally, dogs have no difficulty learning to avoid shock in this situation by leaping a barrier to the other side of the shuttle box. This was the case for the dogs which had previously been given escapable shock while harnessed. However, in phase two, the dogs which had previously been exposed to inescapable shock failed to jump the barrier in the shuttle box to escape from the electric shock. They were described as being initially agitated in reaction to the shock, but, rather than run around "frantically" until they discovered that they could escape the shock by leaping the barrier, they would sit or lie down quietly whining; that is, they acted as if they were "helpless" and incapable of escaping. The interpretation was that the earlier experience with inescapable shock had made them unable to cope with the present situation. One theory to explain these data was that the dogs learned during the initial experience that outcomes were not contingent on their behavior; that is, they learned to be helpless.

To reverse this state, attempts were made to retrain the dogs by trying to coax them across the barrier. This was very difficult, and ultimately it was found that the only effective way was to forcibly drag the dogs across the barrier and thus terminate the shock. This was not easy to do, and it took many such efforts before most of the dogs "learned" this response enough to do it by themselves. However, with this method, it was eventually possible to rehabilitate them.

The subsequent literature on learned helplessness is enormous and, as in the case of separation models, controversial (February, 1978 Special Issue of *Journal of Abnormal Psychology* Huesmann, ed. Literally thousands of articles have been written on this topic as graduate students and other workers studied the effect of changing one variable or another. Controversies have included such issues as the degree of motivational deficit, the role of motor requirements, the role of cognitive deficits in these animals, and the relationship with subtypes of depression. These are, by and large, highly technical debates and, although relevant, impossible to incorporate in any detail here. Part of the confusion and controversy with the term *learned helplessness* comes from the fact that it has been used in many different ways. Maier (1984) has pointed out that the term has been used to refer to a particular behavioral phenomenon, to a general category of effects, and to a theoretical position. Maier feels that the common, core concept involves the controllability of events and that this is central to all the other uses. In other words, the term refers to situations where the effects are produced by the uncontrollable nature of events rather than by the events themselves. There seems to be general consensus that the factor of uncontrollability is key in producing major behavioral and neurobiological effects. However, there is considerable controversy regarding whether it is necessary to invoke cognition or learning to explain the results of studies in which subjects have no control over events.

For example, Weiss and group (Weiss and Goodman, 1984; Weiss, Glazer, and Pohorecky, 1976; Weiss, Glazer, Pohorecky, Bailey, Schneider, 1979; Weiss, Goodman, Ambrose, Webster, and Hoffman, 1984) initially offered the "motor activation" hypothesis to explain the results of uncontrollability experiments. This hypothesis stated that the changes seen in such experiments were caused by disturbances of norepinephrine (NE) in the brain, and indeed, if the changes in NE, which are seen in uncontrollability experiments, were prevented by prior pharmacological treatments, the behavioral effects did not occur. In later studies of what Weiss calls "stress-induced depression" (Weiss, Goodman, Ambrose, Webster, and Hoffman, 1984), rats were exposed to strong, uncontrollable shocks after which they showed "depressed" behavior. The symptomatology produced by uncontrollable shock included such things as decreased food and/or water consumption, weight loss, poor performance in tasks requiring active motor behavior, loss of normal aggressiveness or competitiveness, loss of normal grooming or play activity, and decreased sleep.

There are now considerable data from a systematic series of studies to show that this stress-induced depression is caused by significant depletion of NE in the locus coeruleus region of the brain stem (Weiss and

Goodman, 1984). Based on the above body of work, it has been argued that the uncontrollability effects can be completely explained in neurochemical terms, and it is not necessary to invoke any cognitive or learning concepts implied by the term *learned* helplessness.

Though there are a number of methodological differences between the work of Weiss's group and the originators of the learned helplessness hypothesis, the central importance of uncontrollability seems to hold up. However, as stated above, there are significant interpretative differences around the issue of whether it is necessary to use cognitive or learning explanations to explain the results of uncontrollability studies. The argument has been presented that since inescapable shock is simply a more severe stressor than escapable shock and thus has more neurobiological effects, a cognitive or learning interpretation is unnecessary.

It is probable—and Maier (1984) has also expressed a variant of this position—that we are talking about different levels of analyses rather than competing theories, though the dialogue has often taken the latter form. The fact that there are well-substantiated neurobiological changes associated with stress-induced depression models involving uncontrollability does not invalidate psychological explanations, anymore than psychological explanations exclude underlying, and probably necessary, neurochemistry. The presence of a required NE deficit does not invalidate the behavioral phenomenon. It merely substantiates the presence of an important neurochemical substrate, the presence of which does not mean that a cognitive deficit may not also exist. Indeed, this is probably the most exciting aspect of this particular research area, namely, that a clearly behaviorally induced state is associated with major changes in certain neurobiological systems, and that if these changes can be prevented, the behavioral state does not develop. Likewise, the behavioral state can be forestalled or reversed with certain behavioral manipulations. It would be interesting to know if behavioral reversal of the syndrome also leads to reversal of the biological changes or if reversal of the biological changes alone, once the syndrome is set in motion, reverses the behavioral aspects. We know that in many cases of human depression all of the significant behavioral and cognitive changes in depression are not necessarily reversed with drugs that presumably "fix" some underlying biological alterations. At times, as with the underlying neurochemistry, the altered cognitions and behaviors must be dealt with directly. The exciting finding of a complex interplay between a cognitive–behavioral state and neurobiology clearly warrants further investigation.

There is other exciting work going on in the uncontrollability area that relates mainly to this interface between the behavioral state and underlying neurochemical substrates. In addition to the work by Weiss's group mentioned previously, other major groups involved have been Anisman; Henn, Petty, and Sherman; and Maier.

Anisman and colleagues (Anisman, Irwin, and Sklar, 1979; Anisman, Remington, and Sklar, 1979; Anisman, Grimmer, Irwin, Remington, and Sklar, 1979; Anisman, Suissa, and Sklar, 1980; Anisman, Pizzino, and Sklar, 1980; Anisman and Zacharko, 1982), like Weiss, found an NE depletion in mice exposed to inescapable shock but not in mice allowed to escape during pretreatment. They also think that NE is mainly responsible for later escape deficits in yoked animals. One of their important findings is that transient NE depletion produced by inescapable shock can later be provoked by only moderate shock. The question of what happens to NE levels with chronic (vs acute) exposure to inescapable shock, and the relationship of this to subsequent interference effects is controversial. Even if levels of NE returned to normal, it is still possible, in this paradigm, that there have been hyposensitive receptors produced. This controversy provides an appropriate case for the use of animal models to examine the behavioral–neurobiological interface.

Pharmacological agents have also been studied in the learned helplessness models. In general, the behavioral syndrome can be treated with tricyclic antidepressants, atypical antidepressants, or monoamine oxidase inhibitors. Treatment with antipsychotics, anxiolytics, stimulants, or sedative drugs is ineffective. There are also reports of reversal by Dopa, vasopressin, antiserum, apomorphine, and clonidine, although the behavioral paradigms are not exactly the same.

Petty and Sherman (Petty and Sherman, 1980, 1981a, 1981b; Sherman and Petty, 1980, 1982) have also studied the neurochemical specificity of the learned helplessness paradigm. They have reported that hippocampal *in vitro* release of gamma aminobutyric acid (GABA) decreases in helpless animals, and that treatment with imipramine or iprindole increases GABA flux through the neuronal pool in the hippocampus. The neurochemical and behavioral effects appear to be highly related to the amount of drug present in the neocortex. Furthermore, they have reported that helplessness can be prevented by fornix transection or cortical lesions and is made worse by hippocampectomy. It can be reversed by pharmacological and/or neurochemical stimulation of the cortex, hippocampus, or septum, with significant regional specificity. Table 4 summarizes some of the key aspects of uncontrollability models.

In summary, experimental models involving induction of uncontrollability have now been described in a variety of species—dogs, mice, rats, pigeons, fish, and maybe humans, although, in the case of hu-

Table 4 Uncontrollability Models

Basic paradigm: Exposure to inescapable shock

Behavioral effects: Impaired responding when exposed to escapable shock

Explanations
    1. Cognitive—learned helplessness
    2. Motor activation—motor requirements
    3. Neurobiological—changes in norepinephrine in locus coeruleus
Neurobiological substrates
    1. Norepinephrine depletion
    2. Decreased release of hippocampal gamma aminobutyric acid (GABA)
Treatment influences
    1. Prevented by fornix transection or cortical lesions
    2. Worsened by hippocampectomy
    3. Reversal by pharmacological and/or neurochemical stimulation of cortex, hippocampus, or septum
    4. Treated with:
       tricyclic antidepressants
       atypical antidepressants
       monoamine oxidase inhibitors
    5. Ineffective treatments:
       anxiolytics
       stimulants
       sedative drugs

---

mans, it has been necessary to develop a reformulated version of the hypothesis (Abramson, Seligman, and Teasdale, 1978). There is controversy regarding the interpretation of the data from uncontrollability studies. This centers about the role of underlying neurochemical changes as a sufficient explanation for the behavioral phenomenon, and to what extent it is appropriate and/or necessary to invoke cognitive explanations such as implied in the term *learned* helplessness. Likewise, the theoretical implications of these lines of investigations for subtypes of human depression deserve additional consideration. It seems to me that this paradigm, like separation studies, rather than modeling any specific type of depression, provides another experimental system in animals for investigation of the complex interplay between neurobiology and behavior. As such, the implications extend well beyond any debates about its validity as a general model of depression. These are essentially irresolvable, and perhaps inappropriate, questions, since there is no such thing as a general animal model of depression. However, chronic or acute exposure to uncontrollable events is an important aspect of human functioning. The interaction of prior personality (temperament) and neurobiological functioning with such exposure is undoubtedly important in many forms of psychopathology. Said another way, exposure to uncontrollable, stressful events may be a risk factor in human psychopathology and is one that can usefully be investigated in experimental systems in animals. If our horizons regarding the learned helplessness models can thus be expanded, the usefulness of this approach will be greatly enhanced.

Chronic Stress Models

This is an interesting newer model developed largely in rats by Katz and associates (Katz, 1981a, 1981b, 1982; Katz, Roth, and Carroll, 1981; Katz, Roth, and Schmaltz, 1981; Katz and Hersh, 1981; Katz and Baldrighi, 1982; Katz, Roth, Metford, Carroll, and Barchas, 1982; Roth and Katz, 1981). Basically, in this paradigm, rats are subjected to a chronic stress regimen designed to be unpredictable with regard to the stimulus properties of the stress as well as the time of stress delivery. Stressors are administered over a period of 21 days separated from each other by 1 to 2 days. They are administered at various points in the circadian cycle. Stressors have included switching cagemates, removal from double housing to single housing for 24 hours, 30 minutes of scrambled unpredictable footshock, 46 hours of food or water deprivation, a cold-water swim, shaker stress, and tail pinch. After 21 days of exposure to these stressors, the animals are tested in an open-field test in which they show lowered open-field activity and a failure to show the activation normally seen after an acute stress. The decreased exploratory behaviors are reversed by electroconvulsive treatments and a variety of drugs including monoamine oxidase inhibitors and tricyclic antidepressants. Amphetamine and scopolamine are ineffective. To date, neurobiological studies have not yet been published, but the paradigm does seem to have good pharmacological specificity and could potentially be used for mechanism studies. The major issues raised about this approach concern the severity of the induction techniques; however, as mentioned in earlier chapters, if one wishes to use this kind of paradigm for pharmacological or empirical validity studies, the induction techniques become a secondary consideration. However, this approach emphasizes the combined influence of chronicity and unpredictability in producing behavioral alterations.

Changes in Dominance Hierarchy

Another type of proposed model is based on the importance of dominance in the relationships of most nonhuman primates (Price, 1967). It has been postulated that changes in the stability of the dominance arrangement produce behavioral alterations. Specifically, Price has proposed that the behavioral state associated with advancing in the hierarchy may be elation, and that associated with falling in dominance rank, depression. In this theory, depression is considered to be adaptive, since it prevents the descending animal from fighting back. Price speculates that if this is so, depression could be induced by experimentally altering the dominance hierarchy in some nonhuman primates. Not much research has been done to evaluate this theory, and the evidence for particular behavior patterns occurring in association with specific changes in the hierarchy is fragmentary. Dominance hierarchies are not easy to control in the first place, although recent pioneering work from McGuire concerning dominance and serotonin metabolism in vervet monkeys is interesting in this regard. This work involves manipulation of the dominance hierarchy, careful behavioral observations, and study of the serotonin system. It appears that dominant male adult monkeys have blood serotonin concentrations approximately twice those of subordinate adult males. Furthermore, this is a state-related characteristic that reflects being in the dominant male social position. Spontaneous or experimentally induced changes in social status are accompanied by corresponding increases or decreases in whole blood serotonin concentrations (Raleigh, McGuire, Brammer, and Yuwiler, 1984). It will be interesting to learn about the relationship among social status, other neurotransmitter systems, and social behavior.

Intracranial Self-Stimulation Models

Another proposed animal model of depression is the reward-reduction model using self-stimulating animals. The involvement of catecholamines in the mediation of intracranial self-stimulation (ICSS) has been well established, although there is controversy regarding their relative importance (Crow, 1971; Franklin and Herberg, 1977; German and Bowden, 1974; Herberg, Stephens, and Franklin, 1976; Stein, 1968). In general, agents which enhance the effects of catecholamines tend to increase ICSS responding, while those which impair catecholamine actions tend to depress ICSS response rates. The actions of tricyclics ap-

pear anomalous in this model since they do not enhance ICSS responding despite their well-documented antidepressant action and their
effects on catecholamine systems. Rather, they tend to decrease the rate
of responding and to raise the reward threshold. In view of this, attempts have been made to find an animal model in which tricyclics
potentiate ICSS responding. One such model has been suggested by
Wauquier (1976), who reported that in a situation involving progressive
fixed ratio schedules (i.e., where reinforcement required more and more
effort), antidepressants enhanced responding that otherwise would
have dropped gradually to zero. However, efforts to replicate this work
by Binks *et al.* (1972) were unsuccessful. They trained rats that had
electrodes chronically implanted in the medial forebrain bundle, in progressively increasing fixed ratio schedules. Two tricyclic antidepressants, imipramine and protriptyline, were given, but neither resulted in
response enhancement. Thus this reward-reduction model remains in
question, and much more research is needed regarding the role of ICSS
on a spectrum of approaches to studying specific aspects of depression
in experimental systems in animals. It is worth pursuing, however, in
view of the finding of anhedonia as a key feature in many cases of severe
depression. It would be helpful to have some experimental systems in
which to do some mechanism and pharmacologic studies of this important sign.

Conditioned Motionlessness

Takahashi *et al.* (1974) have proposed an animal model of depression in rats involving pairing a buzzer (conditioned stimulus) with a
tetrabenazine injection (unconditioned stimulus) for at least 11 trials.
Following this kind of conditioning, some rats became motionless after
the presentation of the buzzer alone. It has been reported that this
conditioned motionlessness is associated with an excess of functional
serotonin at the synaptic cleft. The unconditioned motionlessness seen
after tetrabenazine alone is not blocked by imipramine. However, the
conditioned motionlessness is reversed by imipramine and the biochemical data then resemble that of control subjects.

Behavioral Despair

An interesting model developed by Porsolt largely in rats or mice is
called the behavioral despair test (Porsolt, 1981; Porsolt, Anton, Blavel,

and Jalfre, 1977). It is based on the observation that when rats or mice are forced to swim in a restricted space from which they cannot escape, they eventually cease attempts to escape and become immobile. It has been suggested that this characteristic behavioral immobility reflects a state of despair in rats or mice. The immobility is also reduced by non-pharmacological treatments such as electroconvulsive shock, REM sleep deprivation, or even exposure to an enriched environment. It is also reduced by most clinically active antidepressants including the atypical ones. The effects can be seen to a certain extent after acute administration, but greater effects are seen at lower doses after repeated treatments. The drug effect cannot be accounted for simply by saying they increase motor activity, since the doses used generally decrease motor activity. Antidepressants prolong the escape-directed behavior observed at the beginning of a test session, whereas psychostimulants or anti-cholinergics cause a generalized behavioral stimulation. These potential false positives can be distinguished from the effects of true antidepressants. Reported false positives include antihistamines, subconvulsant doses of convulsants, and some neuropeptides. False negatives include clomipramine in rats and salbutanol in rats and mice.

This model was developed mainly for drug screening and thus must be evaluated in terms of its empirical validity, which seems as good as, if not better than, most drug-screening models. At a theoretical level, it has been proposed to be related to the learned helplessness or uncontrollability models. Mechanism studies remain to be done.

Animal Models for Mania

Although there is extensive work targeted toward the development and study of animal models for depression, the amount of work directed toward the development of models for mania is far more limited. However, there is some work, and it is reviewed in this section. The reader is also referred to several recent reviews of this topic for more detail (Harrison-Reed, 1981; Mamelak, 1978; Murphy, 1977; Petty and Sherman, 1981).

It is interesting that there is so little work on mania, because mania, as a clinical syndrome, probably has more clearly described, and clinically agreed upon, behaviors than most psychiatric syndromes. The symptoms of mania are well known and include such things as increased motor and verbal activity, distractibility, lack of need for sleep, labile affective state, increased, but frantic, social activity, increased ag-

Table 5 Antagonism by Lithium of Drug-Induced States in Animals and Man[a]

	Lithium effect	
State	Man	Animals
Amphetamine (low dose) Hyperactivity, activation	Blocked	Reduced
Amphetamine (high dose) Stereotypic behavior	Unchanged or prolonged	—
Morphine Excitement, euphoria	Reduced or unchanged	Unchanged
DMI plus tetrabenazine Hyperactivity	Reduced or unchanged	—
L-Dopa Hyperactivity, hypomania	—	Possibly reduced
Ethanol "High"	—	Unchanged
MAO-inhibitor Hyperactivity	Enhanced	—

[a]From Murphy, 1977.

gressive and/or sexual activity, impaired judgment, and disorders of impulse control. There may be delusional thinking, hallucinations, and confusion. Mania tends to run in families, but the pattern of inheritance or genetic mechanisms is still unclear. The underlying mechanisms are essentially unknown, although a variety of neurotransmitter alterations have been suggested. None has been firmly documented at the present time, though active research in this area continues. The syndrome is highly, though not always, responsive to lithium treatment.

Virtually all proposed animal models for mania involve drug induction of various behavioral changes. The main behavioral change usually assessed is hyperactivity. A summary of some of the drug-induced states in animals along with the effects of lithium in animals and man is shown in Table 5.

Amphetamine-Induced Hyperactivity

One proposed animal model of mania involves the administration of low doses of d-amphetamine, sometimes along with chlordiazepoxide (Davies *et al.*, 1974; Dorr *et al.*, 1971; Randrup and Munkvad, 1967; Rushton and Steinberg, 1963, 1966; Steinberg, 1973; Steinberg and

Tomkiewicz 1970). This produces a state of hyperactivity which has been described as "fast and coordinated" and interpreted as "activity for activity's sake." It has been contrasted with the stereotyped activity induced by larger doses of amphetamine (e.g., sniffing, gnawing, head shaking and other small movements). The latter has been proposed as an animal model of schizophrenia. Lithium blocks the effects produced by low-dose amphetamine, (i.e., the hyperactivity and general activation), but has either no effects or actually prolongs the stereotypic behaviors produced by high-dose amphetamine.

Morphine

Morphine activation has also been proposed as an animal model of mania (Carroll and Sharp, 1971). Morphine sulfate (25 mg/kg) has been reported to induce behavioral activation in mice. This has been labeled "intense stereotyped hyperactivity." There are data to suggest that a variety of drugs (e.g., chlorpromazine, haloperidol, cinanserin, methysergide, alpha-methyl-paratyrosine, and para-chlorophenylalanine) will reduce morphine-induced activation. Lithium's effect in this experimental system has not been clear. However, in other experimental systems using morphine, there are reports of lithium's effectiveness. For example, lithium reduces morphine self-administration (Tomkiewicz and Steinberg, 1972) as well as morphine enhanced self-stimulation, using electrodes in the substantia nigra of rats (Liebman and Segal, 1976).

Other Drug-Induced Behaviors

A number of other drugs have been used to induce hyperactivity in animals and studies done of the effectiveness of lithium and/or other drugs in counteracting the activating effects. These include the combination of desmethyl imipramine (DMI) and tetrabenazine, monoamine oxidase (MAO) inhibitors, L-dopa, and ethanol. The effects of lithium on these various drug-induced changes is summarized in Table 5.

Non-Drug–Induced Behaviors in Relation to Models of Mania

The general consensus seems to be that lithium treatment alone, even in doses which block some of the drug effects described above, has little effect on the basal level of spontaneous behavior of animals. However, it should be remembered that the introduction of lithium into clinical psychiatry originated with the observation of Cade (1949) that lithium-treated guinea pigs appeared lethargic. This led to the suggestion that lithium might have antimanic activity. Murphy (1977) has reviewed a scattered literature regarding the possible effects of lithium on baseline behaviors of animals, but none of these effects has actually been related to the concept of animal models of mania as the above studies have.

6-Hydroxydopamine Models of Mania

Another approach used to study mania in animals involves the intraventricular injection of 6-hydroxydopamine (Petty and Sherman, 1981b). An experimental neurotoxin, 6-hydroxydopamine has been reported to produce a permanent and selective depletion of norepinephrine, although the degree of specificity is debated (Bloom *et al.*, 1969; Breese and Traylor, 1970). Sherman and Petty have reported that the intraventricular injection of 6-hydroxydopamine in rats makes them hyperirritable and hyperresponsive to environmental stimuli. The stimulus used in this paradigm was footshock. Animals receiving no treatment other than 6-hydroxydopamine became progressively more hyperresponsive to shock, and, by Day 6, reactivity scores were 67% higher than on Day 0. This pattern of responding did not occur in animals treated with lithium. Instead of a progressive increase in responsiveness to shock, these animals became less responsive and by Day 6 were not different than controls. Actually, by Day 4 they were significantly less reactive to shock than were animals receiving saline. Chronic lithium administration thus prevented the development of hyperreactivity to mild footshock that typically follows 6-hxdroxydopamine injections. However, the effects are not specific to lithium in that animals receiving chlorpromazine after 6-hydroxydopamine were also less hyperreactive, and their behavior was similar to animals receiving lithium. Imipramine had no additional effects over those produced bx 6-hydroxydopamine treatment alone.

In summary, most proposed animal models of mania involve drug precipitation of hyperactivity and evaluation of the effect of lithium and other drugs in reversing this syndrome. Thus, a model's validity in this context has been mainly evaluated by how well lithium works in counteracting the induced behavioral changes and by how specific its effects are. It is important to consider how we might develop additional paradigms for studying mania in animals. Since we know virtually nothing about the etiology of human mania, it is difficult to create a model on the basis of a specific etiology. Indeed, even testable theories are lacking in this area. One intriguing area concerns the role of circadian and other biological rhythms and to what extent alterations in biological clocks might be important factors in mania. Certain animal species might lend themselves to experimental manipulation of bodily rhythms and to the study of behavioral and biological consequences along with the effects of lithium, which is now known to affect such rhythms. Since mania seems to be, in part, heavily genetically determined, the question of selective breeding for one or another cluster of symptoms also needs to be considered.

Some of the newer thinking in this area is represented in a recent article by Gardner (1982) in which he presented an evolutionary model of manic–depressive disorder. This model has the following major elements as presented by Gardner:

1. Manic and depressive behaviors are evidence of triggered fundamental alpha and omega states of social rank and are not by themselves pathologic.
2. What is pathologic is their tendency to be stimulated too easily and maintained too rigidly because of an unstable component in the susceptible person's neural organization.
3. For mania, at least, psychotic consequences may stem from a positive-feedback cycle in the person imbued with an inappropriate alpha state, who reacts with primitive defenses to feedback that are contrary to his sense of state.
4. Ease of onset and resistance to offset stimuli may be separable features of manic–depressive disorder.

Basically, this evolutionary model proposes that mania and depression are not states peculiar to humans but are universal in social animals and are related to rigidity of alpha- and omega-type behaviors which occur out of context. This interesting theoretical conceptualization has a number of research implications for the possible development of animal models of mania. These implications include the possibility that animal strains could be bred to exhibit behaviors characteristic of extreme alpha or omega states with minimal provocation. Also, might it be possible to produce a dissociation between an animal's social role and state? These and other implications have been developed in more detail by Gardner in his important theoretical article regarding new evolutionary perspectives on developing experimental systems in which to study mania.

Summary of Key Points

- *Scattered anecdotal case reports dating back to the 1920s suggest that animals could show behavioral changes resembling those seen in human depression.*

- *The controlled, laboratory study of animal models of depression dates to the 1960s and has experienced a very rapid growth since that time.*

- *The major approaches used to develop animal models of human depression can be categorized as follows: (a) pharmacological, (b) separation, (c) uncontrollability (learned helplessness), (d) imposition of multiple stressors and conflict, and (e) alteration of dominance patterns.*

- *Depression is a complex and multivariate illness. There is probably a psychobiological final common pathway with numerous variables influencing whether or not depressions develop as well as the form of the depression. These influencing variables include genetic, developmental, interpersonal, personality, social, and physiological factors.*

- *Given such a complex and multivariate illness, it becomes especially important to have experimental systems in which to do controlled, prospective studies. Animal models represent one approach to this problem. Thus, the animal work has clinical implications in helping to sort out how each of these variables individually can potentially influence the development of depressive behaviors and how they might interact.*

- *Pharmacologically induced models have been, and continue to be, important clinically in terms of screening clinically effective drugs. None is perfect, in the sense that there are false positives and false negatives, but these models are an aspect of animal modeling that have had clinical relevance in terms of helping to develop a broader range of effective antidepressant medications.*

- *Separation studies in animals have represented another approach to animal modeling. They have documented, in a systematic way, the powerful effects of disrupting attachment systems and have helped in the formulation of theories of attachment which are now part of the fabric of general, and especially child, psychiatry. Specifically, this category of studies has also provided empirical support for the long-term effects of early losses and for the potential neurobiological impact of such experiences.*

- *Animal studies of uncontrollability (learned helplessness models) have also had clinical implications regardless of debates about their interpretation. They have documented the significant effects on animals of continued experiences with being unable to control what happens. The link-*

age of this line of animal work with cognitive theories of depression has been a close one, and it has led to new approaches in our conceptualization of certain aspects of depressions and to some of the cognitive therapies. Continuing work with the neurobiological substrates of uncontrollability are likely to further help us understand this interaction.

- *Chronic stress models emphasize the combined influence of chronicity and unpredictability in producing behavioral alterations that have some similiarity to those seen in depression and are altered by the same treatments that help in human depression. Certainly, the issues of chronicity and unpredictability are ones that clinicians are aware of, and there are now animal paradigms for providing specific empirical data about their effects.*
- *The possible role of dominance hierarchy changes in relationship to depression and mania represents another approach to animal modeling that has obvious clinical implications. Thus far, the data are limited, but this may be an area in which to follow future developments.*
- *A very limited amount of work has been done on animal models of mania. The approaches mainly involve drug induction of hyperactivity and evaluation of the effects of lithium. An evolutionary model of manic–depressive disorder has been recently presented that may help guide some future research in this area.*

References

Abramson, L. Y., Seligman, M. E. P., and Teasdale, J. D. (1978) Learned Helplessness in Humans: Critique and Reformulation. *Journal of Abnormal Psychology* **87(1):** 49–74.

Ackerman, S. H., Hofer, M. A., and Weiner, H. (1979) Sleep and Temperature Regulation During Restraint Stress in Rats Is Affected by Prior Maternal Separation. *Psychosomatic Medicine* **41:** 311–319.

Akiskal, H. S., and McKinney, W. T. (1973) Depressive Disorders: Toward a Unified Hypothesis. *Science* **182:** 20–29.

Akiskal, H. S., and McKinney, W. T. (1975) Overview of Recent Research in Depression: Integration of Ten Conceptual Models Into a Comprehensive Clinical Frame. *Archives of General Psychiatry32:* 285–305.

Akiskal, H. S., Bitar, A. H., Puzantian, V. R., Rosenthal, T. L., and Walker, P. W. (1978) The Nosological Status of Neurotic Depression: A Prospective Three to Four Year Examination in Light of the Primary-Secondary and Unipolar-Bipolar Dichotomies. *Archives of General Psychiatry* **35:** 756–766.

Anisman, H., and Zacharko, R. M. (1982) Depression: The Predisposing Influence of Stress. *Behavioral and Brain Science* **5:** 89–137.

Anisman, J., Grimmer, L., Irwin, J., Remington, G., and Sklar, L. S. (1979) Escape Performance After Inescapable Shock in Select Bred Lines of Mice: Response Maintenance and Catecholamine Act *Journal of Comparative and Physiological Psychology* **93:** 229–241.

Anisman, H., Remington, G., and Sklar, L. (1979) Effect of Inescapable Shock on Subsequent Escape Performance: Catecholaminergic and Cholinergic Mediation of Response Initiation and Maintenance. *Psychopharmacology* **61**: 107–124.

Anisman, H., Irwin, J., and Sklar, L. (1979) Deficits of Escape Performance Following Catecholaminergic Depletion: Implications for Behavioral Deficits Induced by Uncontrollable Stress. *Psychopharmacology* **64**: 163–170(a).

Anisman, H., Pizzino, A. and Sklar, L. S. (1980) Coping With Stress, Norepinephrine Depletion, and Escape Performance. *Brain Research* **191**: 583–588.

Anisman, H., Suissa, A., and Sklar, L. S. (1980) Escape Deficits Induced by Uncontrollable Stress: Antagonism by Dopamine and Norepinephrine Agonists. *Behavioral and Neural Biology* **28**: 34–47.

Babington, R. G. (1977) The Pharmacology of Kindling. In *Animal Models in Psychiatry and Neurology*, I. Hanin and E. Usdin (Eds.). Oxford: Pergamon Press.

Beck, A. (1967) *Depression: Clinical, Experimental and Theoretical Aspects.* New York: Harper and Row.

Binks, S. M., Murchie, J. K., and Greenwood, D. T. (1979) A Reward–Reduction Model of Depression Using Self-Stimulating Rats: An Appraisal. *Pharmacology, Biochemistry, and Behavior* **10**: 441–443.

Bloom, F. E., Algeri, S., Gropetti, A., Revuelta, A., and Costa, E. (1969) Lesions of Central Norepinephrine Terminals With 6-Hydroxydopamine: Biochemistry and Fine Structure. *Science* **166**: 1284–1286.

Bowden, D. M., and McKinney, W. T. (1972) Behavioral Effects of Peer Separation, Isolation, and Reunion On Adolescent Male Rhesus Monkeys. *Developmental Psychobiology* **5**: 353–362.

Bowlby, J. (1960a) Separation Anxiety. *International Journal of Psychoanalysis* **41**: 89–113.

Bowlby, J. (1960b) Grief and Mourning in Infancy and Early Childhood. *Psychoanalytic Study of the Child* **15**: 9–52.

Bowlby, J. (1961) Processes of Mourning. *International Journal of Psychoanalysis* **42**: 317–340.

Breese, G. R., and Traylor, T. C. (1970) Effect of 6-Hydroxydopamine on Brain Norepinephrine and Dopamine: Evidence for Selective Degeneration of Catecholamine Neurons. *Journal of Pharmacology and Experimental Therapeutics* **174**: 413–420.

Breese, G. P., Smith, R. D., Mueller, R. A., Howard, J. L., Prange, A. J., Lipton, M. A., Young, L. D., McKinney, W. T., and Lewis, J. K. (1973) Induction of Adrenal Catecholamine-Synthesizing Enzymes Following Mother–Infant Separation *Nature: New Biology* **246**: 94–96.

Brown, G. W., Sklar, R., Harris, T. O., and Birley, J. C. T., (1973a) Life Events and Psychiatric Disorders, Part I: Some Methodological Issues. *Psychological Medicine* **3**: 74–87.

Brown, G. W., Harris, T. O., and Peto, J. (1973b) Life Events and Psychiatric Disorders, Part II: Nature of Causal Link. *Psychological Medicine* **3**: 159–176.

Brown, G. W., Nibhrolchain, M., and Harris, T. O. (1979) Psychotic and Neurotic Depression, Part III: Aetiological and Background Factors. *Journal of Affective Disorders* **1**: 195–211.

Bunney, W. E., and Davis, J. (1965) Norepinephrine in Depressive Reactions. *Archives of General Psychiatry* **13**: 483–494.

Cade, J. F. J. (1949) Lithium Salts in Treatment of Psychotic Excitement. *Medical Journal of Australia* **2**: 349–352.

Cairncross, K. D., Cox, B., Forster, C., and Wren, A. F. (1978) A New Model for the Detection of Antidepressant Drugs: Olfactory Bulbectomy in the Rat Compared With Existing Models. *Journal of Pharmacological Methods* **1**: 131–143.

Carroll, B. J., Sharp, P. T. (1971) Rubidium and Lithium: Opposite Effects on Amine-Mediated Excitement. *Science* 172:1355–1357.

Coe, C. L., Mendoza, S. P., Smotherman, W. P., Levine, S. (1978) Mother–Infant Attachment in the Squirrel Monkey: Adrenal Response to Separation. *Behavioral Biology* 22: 256–263.

Coe, C., Wiener, S., Rosenberg, L., and Levine, S. (1985) Endocrine and Immune Responses to Separation and Maternal Loss in Nonhuman Primates. In *The Biology of Social Attachment*, M. Reite and T. Field (Eds.). New York: Academic Press.

Colpaert, F. C., Lenaerts, F. M., Niemegeers, C. J. E., and Janssen, P. A. J. (1975) A Critical Study on RO-4-1284 Antagonism in Mice. *Archives Internationales de Pharmacodynamic et de Therapie* 215: 40–90.

Coppen, A. J. (1968) Depressed States and Indolealkylamines *Advances in Pharmacology #6* New York: Academic Press.

Coppen, A., and Shaw, D. (1963) Mineral Metabolism in Melancholia. *British Medical Journal* 2: 1439–1444.

Coppen, A., Shaw, D., Malleson, S., and Costain, R. (1966) Mineral Metabolism in Mania. *British Medical Journal* 1: 71–75.

Crow, T. J. (1971) The Relationship Between Electrical Self-Stimulation Sites and Catecholamine-Containing Neurones in Rat Mesencephalon. *Experientia* 27: 662.

Davies, C., Sanger, D. J., Steinberg, H., Kiewicz, T., and U'Prichard, D. C. (1974) Lithium and Alpha-methyl-paratyrosine Prevent Manic Activity in Rodents" *Psychopharmacologia* 36: 263.

Delini-Stula, A., Baumann, P., and Buch, O. (1979) Depression of Exploratory Activity by Clonidine in Rats as a Model for the Detection of Relatively Pre- and Postsynaptic Central Noradrenergic Receptor Selectivity of Alpha-adrenolytic Drugs. *Archives of Pharmacology* 307: 115–122.

Dolhinow, P. (1980) An Experimental Study of Mother Loss in the Indian Langur Monkey (*Presbytis entellus*). *Folia Primatologica* 33: 77–128.

Dorr, M., Joyce, D., Porsolt, R. D., Steinberg, H., Summerfield, A., and Tomkiewicz, M. (1971) Persistence of Dose-Related Behavior in Mice" *Nature* 228: 469.

Dubin, R. (1969) *Theory Building*. New York: The Free Press.

Franklin, K. B. J., and Herberg, L. J. (1977) Non-Contingent Displacement of Catecholamines by Intraventricular Tyramine: Biphasic Dose/Response Effects on Self-Stimulation. *Neuropharmacology* 16: 53–55.

Freis, E. D. (1954) Mental Depression in Hypertensive Patients Treated for Long Periods With Large Doses of Reserpine. *New England Journal of Medicine* 251: 1006.

Garattini, S., and Jori, A. (1967) Interactions Between Imipramine-like Drugs and Reserpine on Body Temperature. In *Antidepressant Drugs*, S. Garattini and M. N. G. Dukes (Eds.). Amsterdam: Excerpta Medica Foundation, pp. 179–193.

Gardner, R. (1982) Mechanisms in Manic-Depressive Disorder: An Evolutionary Model. *Archives of General Psychiatry* 39: 1430–1441.

German, D. C., and Bowden, D. M. (1974) Catecholamine Systems As the Neural Substrate for Intracranial Self-Stimulation: A Hypothesis. *Brain Research* 73: 381–419.

Goodwin, F. K., and Bunney, W. E., (1971) Depressions Following Reserpine-A Reevaluation. *Seminars in Psychiatry* 3: 435–438.

Gower, A. J., and Marriott, A. S. (1980) The Inhibition of Clonidine-Induced Sedation in the Mouse by Antidepressant Drugs. *British Journal of Pharmacology* 69: 287–288.

Green, A. R., Head, D. J., Lister, S., and Molyneux, S. (1982) The Effect of Acute and Repeated Desmethylimipramine Administration on Clonidine-Induced Hypoactivity in Rats. *British Journal of Pharmacology* 75: 33.

Harrison-Read, P. E. (1981) Behavioral Studies With Lithium in Rats: Implications for Animal Models of Mania and Depression. In *Neuroendocrine Regulation and Altered Behavior*, L. Radhey, and L. Singa (Eds.). New York: Plenum Press, pp. 223–262.

Hebb, D. O. (1947) Spontaneous Neurosis in Chimpanzees. *Psychosomatic Medicine* 9: 3–16.

Herberg, L. J., Stephens, D. N., and Franklin, K. B. J. (1976) Catecholamines and Self-Stimulation: Evidence Suggesting a Reinforcing Role for Noradrenaline and a Motivating Role for Dopamine. *Pharmacology, Biochemistry, and Behavior* 4: 575–582.

Hinde, R. A., and Davies, L. M. (1972) Changes in Mother–Infant Relationship After Separation in Rhesus Monkeys. *Nature* 239: 41–42.

Hinde, R. A., and Spencer-Booth, Y. (1970) Individual Differences in the Responses of Rhesus Monkeys to a Period of Separation From Their Mothers. *Journal of Child Psychology and Psychiatry* 11: 159–176.

Hinde, R. A., and White, L. E. (1974) Dynamics of a Relationship: Rhesus Mother–Infant Ventro-Ventral Contact. *Journal of Comparative Physiological Psychology* 86: 8–23.

Hinde, R. A., Spencer-Booth, Y., and Bruce, M. (1966) Effects of 6-Day Maternal Deprivation on Rhesus Monkey Infants. *Nature* 210: 1021–1023.

Hoesman, R. L. (guest editor) (1978) Learned Helplessness as a Model of Depression. *Journal of Abnormal Psychology* (special issue) Washington, D.C.: American Psychological Association.

Hofer, M. A. (1970) Physiological Responses of Infant Rats to Separation from Their Mothers. *Science* 168: 871–873.

Hofer, M. A. (1975a) Infant Separation Responses and the Maternal Role. *Biological Psychiatry* 19:149–153.

Hofer, M. A. (1975b) Studies On How Early Separation Produces Behavioral Change in Young Rats. *Psychosomatic Medicine* 37: 245–264.

Hofer, M. A. (1975c) Survival and Recovery of Physiological Functions After Early Maternal Separation in Young Rats. *Physiology and Behavior* 15: 475–480.

Hofer, M. A. (1976) The Organization of Sleep and Wakefulness After Maternal Separation in Young Rats. *Developmental Psychobiology* 9: 189–203.

Howard, J. L., Sorok, F. E., and Cooper, B. R. (1981) Empirical Behavioral Models of Depression, With Emphasis on Tetrabenazine Antagonism. In *Antidepressants: Neurochemical, Behavioral, and Clinical Perspectives*, S. J. Enna, J. B. Malick, E. Richelson (Eds.). New York: Raven Press, pp. 107–120.

Hrdina, P. D, Kulmiz, P. von, and Stretch, R. (1979) Pharmacological Modification of Experimental Depression in Infant Macaques. *Psychopharmacology* 64: 89–93.

Huesmann, L. R., (Ed.) (1978) *Journal of Abnormal Psychology* 87:(1) Special Issue: Learned Helplessness as a Model of Depression.

Hunt, G. E., Atrens, D. M., and Johnson, G. F. S (1981) The Tetracyclic Antidepressant Mianserin: Evaluation of Its Blockade of Presynaptic Alpha-adrenoreceptors in a Self-Stimulation Model Using Clonidine. *European Journal of Pharmacology* 70: 59–63.

Janowsky, D., El-Yousef, K., Davis, J. M., Hubbard, B., and Sekerke, H. (1972) A Cholinergic-Adrenergic Hypothesis of Mania and Depression. *Lancet* 2: 632–635.

Jensen, G. D., and Tolman, C. W. (1962) Mother–Infant Relationship in the Monkey, *Macaca nemestrina:* The Effect of Brief Separation and Mother–Infant Specificity. *Journal of Comparative Physiological Psychology* 55: 131–136.

Kaplan, J. (1970) The Effects of Separation and Reunion on the Behavior of Mother and Infant Squirrel Monkeys. *Developmental Psychobiology* 3: 43–52.

Katz, R. J. (1981a) Animal Model of Depression: Effects of Electroconvulsive Shock Therapy. *Neuroscience and Biobehavioral Reviews* 5: 273–279.

Katz, R. J. (1981b) Animal Models and Human Depressive Disorders. *Neuroscience and Biobehavioral Review* **5**: 231–246.

Katz, R. J. (1982) Animal Model of Depression: Pharmacological Sensitivity of a Hedonic Effect. *Pharmacology, Biochemistry, and Behavior* **16**: 965–969.

Katz, R. J., and Baldrighi, G. (1982) A Further Parametric Study of Imipramine in An Animal Model of Depression. *Pharmacology, Biochemistry, and Behavior* **16**: 969–972.

Katz, R. J. and Hersh, S. (1981) Amitryptyline and Scopolamine in an Animal Model of Depression. *Neuroscience and Biobehavioral Reviews* **5**: 265–273.

Katz, R. J., Roth, K. A., and Carroll, B. J. (1981) Acute and Chronic Stress Effects on Open Field Activity in the Rat: Implications for a Model of Depression. *Neuroscience and Biobehavioral Reviews* **5(2)**: 247–253.

Katz, R. J., Roth, K. A., and Schmaltz, K. (1981) Amphetamine and Tranylcypromine in an Animal Model of Depression: Pharmacological Specifity of the Reversal Effect. *Neuroscience and Biobehavioral Reviews* **5**: 259–265.

Katz, R. J., Roth, K. A., Mefford, I. A., Carroll, B. J., and Barchas, J. (1982) The Chronically Stressed Rat—A Novel Animal Model of Endogenomorphic Depression. *Proceedings of III World Congress of Biological Psychiatry.* Stockholm, Sweden.

Kaufman, I. C., and Rosenblum, L. A. (1967a) Depression in Infant Monkeys Separated From their Mothers. *Science* **155**: 1030–1031.

Kaufman, I. C., and Rosenblum, L. A. (1967b) The Reaction to Separation in Infant Monkeys: Anaclitic Depression and Conservation-Withdrawal. *Psychosomatic Medicine* **29**: 648–675.

Kokkinidis, L., Zacharko, R. M., Predy, P. A. (1980) Post-Amphetamine Depression of Self-Stimulation Responding from the Substantia Nigra: Reversal by Tricyclic Antidepressants. *Pharmacology, Biochemistry, and Behavior* **13**: 379–383.

Kraemer, G. W. (1985) Effects of Differences in Early Social Experience on Primate Neurobiological-Behavioral Development. In: *The Psychobiology of Attachment.* M. Reite, T. Field, (Eds.). New York: Academic Press, pp. 135–161.

Kraemer, G. W., and McKinney, W. T. (1979) Interactions of Pharmacological Agents which Alter Biogenic Amine Metabolism and Depression: An Analysis of Contributing Factors within a Primate Model of Depression. *Journal of Affective Disorders* **1**: 33–54

Kraemer, G. W., Lin, D. H., Moran, E. C., and McKinney, W. T. (1980) Effects of Alcohol on the Despair Response to Peer Separation in Rhesus Monkeys. *Psychopharmacology* **73**: 307–310.

Kraemer, G. W., Ebert, M. H., Lake, R. C., and McKinney, W. T. (1984) Cerebrospinal Fluid Measures of Neurotransmitter Changes Associated with Pharmacological Alteration of the Despair Response to Social Separation in Rhesus Monkeys. *Psychiatry Research* **11**: 303–315.

Lapin, I., and Oxenkrug, G. (1969) Intensification of the Central Serotonergic Process As a Possible Determinant of Thymoleptic Effect. *Lancet* **1**: 132–136.

Levine, S., Coe, C. L., Smotherman, W. P. (1978) Prolonged Cortisol Elevation in the Infant Squirrel Monkey After Reunion With Mother. *Physiology and Behavior* **20**: 7–10.

Lewis, J. K., McKinney, W. T., Young L. D., Kraemer, G. W. (1976) Mother–infant Separation in Rhesus Monkeys as a Model of Human Depression: A Reconsideration. *Archives of General Psychiatry* **33**:699–705.

Liebman, J. M., Segal, D. S. (1976) Lithium Differentially Antagonises Self-Stimulation Facilitated by Morphine and (+)Amphetamine. *Nature* **260(5547)**:161–163.

Limieux, G., Davignon, A., Genst, J. (1956) Depressive States During Rauwolfia Therapy for Arterial Hypertension" *Canadian Medical Assn. Journal* **74**: 522.

Lynch, M. A., and Leonard, B. E. (1978) Effect of Chronic Amphetamine Administration on the Behavior of Rats in the Open Field Apparatus: Reversal of Post-Withdrawal Depression by Two Antidepressants. *J.Pharmacy and Pharmacology* 30: 798–799.

MaLer, S. F. (1984) Learned Helplessness and Animal Models of Depression. *Progress in Neuropsychopharmacology and Biological Psychiatry.*

Mamelak, M. (1978) An Amphetamine Model of Manic Depressive Illness. *International Pharmacopsychiatry* 13: 193–208.

Maxim, P. E. (1980) Rewarding Brain Stimulation and the Peer–Infant Separation Syndrome. *Physiology and Behavior* 25: 53–61.

McKinney, W. T., Suomi, S. J., and Harlow, H. F. (1972) Repetitive Peer Separations of Juvenile-age Rhesus Monkeys. *Archives of General Psychiatry* 27: 200–203.

Mineka, S., and Suomi, S. J. (1978) Social Separation in Monkeys. *Psychological Bulletin* 85: 1376–1400.

Moller-Nielsen, I. (1980) Tricyclic Antidepressants: General Pharmacology. In *Psychotropic Agents. Part I. Antipsychotics and Antidepressants,* F. Hoffmeister and G. Stille (Eds.). Berlin: Springer Verlag, pp. 399–414.

Murphy, D. L. (1977) Animal Models for Mania. In *Animal Models in Psychiatry and Neurology,* I. Hanin and E. Usdin (Eds.). New York: Pergamon Press, pp. 211–223.

Overmier, J. B., Seligman, M. E. (1967) Effects of inescapable Shock upon Subsequent Escape and Avoidance Responding. *Journal of Comparative and Physiological Psychology* 63:28–33.

Panksepp, J., Herman, B., Conner, R., Bishop, P., and Scott, J. P. (1978) The Biology of Social Attachments: Opiates Alleviate Separation Distress. *Biological Psychiatry* 13: 607–618.

Panksepp, J., Vilberg, T., Bean, N. J., Coy, D. H., and Kastin, A. J. (1978) Reduction of Distress Vocalization in Chicks by Opiate-like Peptides. *Brain Research Bulletin* 3: 663–667.

Paykel, E. S. (1974) Recent Life Events and Clinical Depression. In *Life Stress and Illness,* E. K. Gunderson and R. H. Rahe (Eds.). pp. 134–163. Charles C. Thomas: Springfield, IL.

Paykel, E. S. (1978) Contribution of Life Events to Causation of Psychiatric Illness. *Psychological Medicine* 8: 245–253.

Paykel, E. S. (1979a) Causal Relationships Between Clinical Depression and Life Events. In *Stress and Mental Disorder* J. E. Barrett (Ed.). New York: Raven Press.

Paykel, E. S. (1979b) Predictors of Treatment Response. In *Psychopharmacology of Affective Disorders,* E. S. Paykel and A. Coppen (Eds.). Oxford: Oxford University Press, pp. 193–200.

Paykel, E. S. (1982a) Life Events and Early Environment. In *Handbook of Affective Disorders,* E. S. Paykel (Ed.). New York: Churchill Livingstone, pp. 146–161.

Paykel, E. S. (1982b) Recent Life Events. *Proceedings of Dahlem Workshop on The Origins of Depression: Current Concepts and Approaches,* October 31–November 5, 1982.

Pettijohn, T. F. (1979) Attachment and Separation Distress in the Infant Guinea Pig. *Developmental Psychobiology* 12: 73–81.

Pettijohn, T. F., Wong, T. W., Ebert, P. D., and Scott, J. D. (1977) Alleviation of Separation Distress in Three Breeds of Young Dogs. *Developmental Psychobiogy* 10: 373–381.

Petty, F., and Sherman, A. D. (1980) Regional Aspects of the Prevention of Learned Helplessness By Desipramine. *Life Sciences* 26: 1447–1452.

Petty, F., and Sherman, A. D. (1981a) GABAergic Modulation of Learned Helplessness. *Pharmacology, Biochemistry, and Behavior* 15: 567–570.

Petty, F., and Sherman, A. D. (1981b) A Pharmacologically Pertinent Animal Model of Mania. *Journal of Affective Disorders* 3: 381–387.

Porsolt, R. D. (1981) Behavioral Despair. In *Antidepressants: Neurochemical, Behavioral, and Clinical Perspectives*, S. J. Enna, J. B. Malick, E. Richelson (Eds.). New York: Raven Press, pp. 121–139.

Porsolt, R. D. (1982) Pharmacological Models of Depression. *Proceedings of Dahlem Conference on The Origins of Depression: Current Concepts and Approaches*, October 31–November 5, 1982.

Porsolt, R. D., Anton, G., Blavel, N., and Jalfre, M. (1977) Depression: A New Animal Model Sensitive to Antidepressant Treatments. *Nature* **21**: 730–732.

Prange, A. (1964) The Pharmacology and Biochemistry of Depression. *Diseases of the Nervous System* **25**: 217–221.

Price, J. (1967) The Dominance Hierarchy and The Evolution of Mental Illness. *Lancet* **2**: 243–246.

Raleigh, M., McGuire, M. T., Brammer, G. L., and Yuwiler, A. (1984) Social and Environmental Influences on Blood Serotonin Concentrations in Monkeys. *Archives of General Psychiatry* **41**: 405–410.

Randrup, A., and Munkvard, I. (1967) Stereotyped Activities Produced by Amphetamine in Several Animal Species and Man. *Psychopharmacology* **11**: 300.

Reite, M. (1977) Maternal Separation in Monkey Infants: A Model of Depression. In *Animal Models in Psychiatry and Neurology* I. Hanin and E. Usdin (Eds.). New York: Pergamon Press, pp. 127–139.

Reite, M., and Short, R. (1977) Nocturnal Sleep in Isolation Reared Monkeys: Evidence for Environmental Independence. *Developmental Psychobiology* **10**: 555–561.

Reite, M., and Short, R. A. (1978) Nocturnal Sleep in Separated Monkey Infants. *Archives of General Psychiatry* **35**: 1247–1253.

Reite, M., Kaufman, I. C., Pauley, J. D., and Stynes, A. J. (1974) Depression in Infant Monkeys: Physiological Correlates. *Psychosomatic Medicine* **36**: 363–367.

Reite, M., Stynes, A. J., Vaughn, L., Pauley, J. D., and Short, R. A. (1976) Sleep in Infant Monkeys: Normal Values and Behavioral Correlates. *Physiology and Behavior* **16**: 245–251.

Reite, M., Short, R., Kaufman, I. C., Stynes, M. J., and Pauley, J. D. (1978) Heart Rate and Body Temperature in Separated Monkey Infants. *Biological Psychiatry* **13**: 91–105.

Reite, M., Harbeck, R., and Hoffman, A. (1981) Altered Cellular Immune Response Following Peer Separation. *Life Sciences* **29**: 1133–1136.

Reite, M., Short, R., Seiler, C., and Pauley, J. D. (1981) Attachment, Loss, and Depression. *Journal of Child Psychology and Psychiatry* **22**: 141–169.

Reite, M., Seiler, C., Crowley, T. J., Hydinger-Macdonald, M., and Short, R. (1982) Circadian Rhythm Changes Following Maternal Separation. *Chronobiologia* **9**: 1–11.

Richter, C. P. (1957) On The Phenomenon of Sudden Death in Animals and Man. *Psychosomatic Medicine* **19**: 191–197.

Robertson, J., and Bowlby, J. (1952) Responses of Young Children to Separation From Their Mothers. *Cours du Centre International de l'Enfance* **2**: 131–142.

Robertson, J., and Robertson, J. (1971) Young Children in Brief Separation. *Psychoanalytic Study of the Child* **26**: 264–315.

Robson, R. D., Antonaccio, M. J., Saelens, J. K., and Liebman, J. (1978) Antagonism by Mianserin and Classical Alpha-adrenoreceptor Blocking Drugs of Some Cardiovascular and Behavioral Effects of Clonidine. *European Journal of Pharmacology* **47**: 431–442.

Rosenblum, L. A., and Kaufman, I. C. (1968) Variations in Infant Developement and Response to Maternal Loss in Monkeys. *American Journal of Orthopsychiatry* **83**: 418–426.

Rosenthal, T. L., Akiskal, H. S., Scott-Strauss, A., Rosenthal, R. H., and David, M. (1981) Familial and Developmental Factors in Characterological Depressions. *Journal of Affective Disorders* 3: 183–192.

Roth, K. A., and Katz, R. J. (1981) Further Studies on a Novel Animal Model of Depression: Therapeutic Effects of a Tricyclic Antidepressant. *Neuroscience and Biobehavioral Reviews* 5: 253–259.

Rushton, R., and Steinberg, H. (1966) Mutual potentiation of Amphetamine and Amylobarbitone Measured by Activity in Rats. *British Journal of Pharmacology* 21: 295.

Rushton, R., and Steinberg, H. (1966) Combined Effects of Chlordiazepoxide and Dexamphetamine on Activity of Rats in an Unfamiliar Environment. *Nature* 211: 1312.

Sanghvi, I. S., and Gershon, S. (1977) Animal Test Models for Prediction of Clinical Antidepressant Activity. In *Animal Models in Psychiatry and Neurology*, I. Hanin and E. Usdin (Eds.). Oxford: Pergamon Press, pp. 157–171.

Scherschlicht, R., Polc, P., Schneeberger, J., Steiner, M., and Haefely, W. (1982) Selective Suppression of Rapid Eye Movement Sleep (REMS) in Cats by Typical and Atypical Antidepressants. In *Typical and Atypical Antidepressants: Molecular Mechanisms*, E. Costa, and G. Racagni (Eds.). New York: Raven Press, pp. 359–364.

Schildkraut, J. (1965) Catecholamine Hypothesis of Affective Disorders. *American Journal of Psychiatry* 122: 509–522.

Seay, B., Hansen, E., and Harlow, H. F. (1962) Mother–Infant Separation in Monkeys. *Journal of Child Psychology and Psychiatry* 3: 123–132.

Seligman, M. E. P., and Maier, S. F. (1967) Failure to Escape Traumatic Shock. *Journal of Experimental Psychology* 74: 1–9.

Seltzer, V., and Tongre, S. R. (1975) Methylamphetamine Withdrawal As a Model for the Depressive State: Antagonism of Post-Amphetamine Depression by Imipramine. *Journal of Pharmacy and Pharmacology* 27: 16P.

Senay, E. C. (1966) Toward an Animal Model of Depression: A Study of Separation Behavior in Dogs. *Journal of Psychiatric Research* 4: 65–71.

Sherman, A. D., and Petty, F. (1980) Neurochemical Basis of the Action of Antidepressants on Learned helplessness. *Behavioral and Neural Biology* 30: 119–134.

Sherman, A. D., and Petty, F. (1982) Additivity of Neurochemical Changes in Learned Helplessness and Imipramine. *Behavioral and Neural Biology* 35: 344–353.

Smotherman, W. P., Hunt, L. E., McGinnis, L. M., and Levine, S. (1979) Mother–Infant Separation in Group Living Rhesus Macaques: A Hormonal Analysis. *Developmental Psychobiology* 12: 211–217.

Solomon, R. L., Corbit, J. D. (1974) An Opponent-Process Theory of Motivation: I. Temporal Dynamics of Affect. *Psychological Review* 81:119–145.

Spitz, R. A. (1946) Anaclitic Depression: An Inquiry into the Genesis of Psychiatric Conditions in Early Childhood, II. *Psychoanalytic Study of the Child* 2: 313–347.

Stach, R., Lazarova, M. B., and Kacz, D. (1980) The Effects of Antidepressant Drugs on the Seizures Kindled From the Rabbit Amygdala. *Polish Journal of Pharmacology and Pharmacy* 32: 505–512.

Steinberg, H. (1973) Animal Models for Behavioral and Biobehavioral Studies on the Effects of Lithium Salts. *Biochemical Society Transactions* 1: 38.

Steinberg, H., and Tomkiewicz, M. (1970) Animal Behavior Models in Psychopharmacology. In *Chemical Influences On Behaviors*, R. Porter and J. Birch (Eds.). CIBA Foundation Study Group, 35: 199; Churchill: London.

Suomi, S. J. (1976) Factors Affecting Responses to Social Separation in Rhesus Monkeys. In *Animal Models in Human Psychobiology*, G. Serban, and A. Kling (Eds.). New York: Plenum Press, pp. 9–26.

Suomi, S. J., Harlow, H. F., and Domek, C. J. (1970) Effect of Repetitive Infant–Infant Separation of Young Monkeys. *Journal of Abnormal Psychology* **76**: 161–172.

Suomi, S. J., Collins, M. L., and Harlow, H. F. (1973) Effects of Permanent Separation from Mother on Infant Monkeys. *Developmental Psychobiology* **9**: 376–384.

Suomi, S. J., Eisele, C. D., Grady, S. A., and Harlow, H. F. (1975) Depressive Behavior in Adult Monkeys Following Separation from Family Environment. *Journal of Abnormal Psychology* **84**: 576–578.

Suomi, S. J., Collins, M. L., Harlow, H. F., and Ruppenthal, G. C. (1976) Effects of Maternal and Peer Separations on Young Monkeys. *Journal of Child Psychology and Psychiatry* **17**: 101–112.

Suomi, S. J., Seaman, S. F., Lewis, J. K., Delizio, R. D., and McKinney, W. T. (1978) Effects of Imipramine Treatment of Separation Induced Social Disorders in Rhesus Monkeys. *Archives of General Psychiatry* **35**: 321–325.

Takahashi, R., Nagayama, H., Kido, A., and Morita, T. (1974) An Animal Model of Depression. *Biological Psychiatry* **9**: 191–204.

Tinkelpaugh, O. L. (1928) The Self-Mutilation of a Male Macaque Rhesus Monkey. *Journal of Mammalogy* **9**: 293–300.

Tomkiewicz, M., Steinberg, H. (1972) Proceedings: Amylobarbitone Abolishes Social Dominance Hierarchies in Laboratory Rats. *British Journal of Pharmacology* 44:351P.

Van Riezen, H., Schnieden, H., and Wren, A. F. (1977) Olfactory Bulb Ablation in the Rat: Behavioral Changes and their Reversal by Antidepressant Drugs. *British Journal of Pharmacology* **60**: 521–528.

Vogel, J. R. (1975) Antidepressants and Mouse Killing (Muricide) Behavior. In *Industrial Pharmacology: Volume 2: Antidepressants*, S. Fielding, and H. Lal (Eds.). New York: Futura, pp. 99–112.

Vogt, J. L., and Levine, S. (1980) Response of Mother and Infant Squirrel Monkeys to Separation and Disturbance *Physiology and Behavior* **24**: 829–832.

Von Voigtlander, P. F., Von Triezenberg, H. G., Losey, E. G. (1978) Interactions between Clonidine and Antidepressant Drugs: A Method for Identifying Antidepressant-like Agents. *Neuropharmacology* **17**: 375–381.

Wauquier, A. (1976) *Brain Stimulation Reward*. New York: American Elsevier, pp. 123–171.

Weiss, J. M., and Goodman, P. A. (1984) Neurochemical Mechanisms Underlying Stress-Induced Depression. In *Stress and Coping* (Vol. 1), P. McCabe and N. Schneiderman (Eds.). Hillsdale, New Jersey: Lawrence-Erlbaum.

Weiss, J. M., Glazer, H. I., Pohorecky, L. A. (1976) Coping Behavior and Neurochemical Changes: An Alternative Explanation for the Original Learned Helplessness Experiments. In *Animal Models in Human Psychobiology*, G. Serban and A. Kling (Eds.). New York: Plenum, pp. 141–173.

Weiss, J. M., Glazer, H. I., Pohorecky, L. A., Bailey, W. H., and Schneider, L. H. (1979) Coping Behavior and Stress-Induced Behavioral Depression: Studies of the Role of Brain Catecholamines. In *The Psychobiology of the Depressive Disorders*, Richard A. Depue (ed.). New York: Academic Press, pp. 125–160.

Weiss, J. M., Goodman, P., Ambrose, M. J., Webster, A., and Hoffman, L. J. (1984) Neurochemical Basis of Behavioral Depression. In *Advances in Behavioral Medicine* (Vol. 1), E. Katkin and S. Manuck (Eds.). Greenwich, Connecticut: JAI Press.

Whybrow, P., and Mendels, J. (1969) Toward a Biology of Depression: Some Suggestions from Neurophysiology. *American Journal of Psychiatry* **125**: 45–54.

Whybrow, P., and Parlatore, A. (1973) Melancholia: A Model in Madness: A Discussion of

Recent Psychobiologic Research Into Depressive Illness. *International Journal of Psychiatry in Medicine* **4**: 351–378.

Whybrow, P., Akiskal, H., and McKinney, W. (1984) *Mood Disorders: Toward a New Psychobiology.* New York: Plenum.

Yerkes, R. M., and Yerkes, A. W. (1929) *The Great Apes.* New Haven: Yale Universities Press.

Animal Models for Anxiety Disorders

Introduction

Anxiety disorders, including panic attacks, are ancient disorders which had been well described prior to *DSM-III* and more recent writers. As part of the rediscovery of this set of disorders, we are in the process of emphasizing their neurobiological aspects and discovering newer ways of treating them with psychopharmacological and/or behavioral means. Studies of the developmental and social origins of anxiety disorders have, unfortunately, become a lower priority item.

It is well known to clinicians that anxiety can be either a symptom or a specific syndrome. The literature to be reviewed on animal models is often very confusing in this regard. In some work anxiety seems to be synonymous with neurosis while in other paradigms what is being studied seems more akin to fear or, on the other hand, to certain kinds of learning behavior. As in the case of the other clinical syndromes used as examples in this book, it is important to keep in mind the core features of the human syndrome.

In the case of anxiety we are, in essence, left with evaluating proposed models by how well they behaviorally resemble human anxiety and by treatment responsiveness criteria. Neither alone is completely satisfactory, but we do not yet know enough about the etiology, pathogenesis, or mechanisms of human anxiety to use these as validating criteria for animal models. As a matter of fact, some of the proposed animal models of anxiety may help clarify some of these issues.

The largest number of approaches to animal modeling of anxiety are based on various versions of operant conditioning paradigms, and validity is evaluated on an empirical basis; namely, how well do clinically effective antianxiety agents work in the paradigms and how specific is the response. In general, a number of the approaches have high empirical validity. This does not necessarily mean that they bear any relationship to the etiology or pathogenesis of human anxiety but still may have merit in the context of this aspect of animal modeling.

Additional models are based on alteration of locus coeruleus function, while another model has been proposed based on studies of invertebrates.

It will be apparent that this area of animal modeling research is also just beginning and that a considerable amount of work is yet to be done. It is hoped, however, that by examining what has been done, some of the general points made in earlier chapters will be illustrated.

Clinical Context

> Fear, rage, and pain, and the pangs of hunger are all primitive experiences which human beings share with the lower animals. These experiences are properly classed as among the most powerful that determine the action of men and beasts. A knowledge of the conditions which attend these experiences, therefore, is of general and fundamental importance in the interpretation of behavior. (Cannon, 1929)

Of the various forms of psychopathology dealt with in this book, this one, surprisingly, requires the most clinical background before a discussion of the specific approaches to developing animal models can be fruitful. As with all types of modeling, it is necessary to understand what is being modeled and for what purpose; only in this context can a model of anxiety be properly evaluated. As will be apparent, most animal modeling work involves the study of animals reacting to external threats, conflicts, trauma, etc. In this historical context, fear and/or learning are probably being modeled more than anxiety. *Anxiety* is a term used to loosely denote a symptom, an emotion, a state of mind or an inferred theoretical construct. It is such a ubiquitous term that there is a danger in hinking we understand it more than we actually do. Anxiety is an important area in which to develop some experimental systems for study.

The concepts of anxiety in general, and of animal models in particular, are being rejuggled so as once again to be in a formative period. This chapter can provide only a very brief review of those aspects which are particularly important to understand in relation to proposed animal models of anxiety.

From a diagnostic standpoint, the anxiety disorders according to *DSM-III* (Diagnostic and Statistical Manual of the American Psychiatric Association, 1980) consist of the following entities:

1. Phobic disorders
2. Anxiety states (anxiety neuroses)
   a. Panic disorder
   b. General anxiety disorder
3. Obsessive–compulsive disorder (or obsessive–compulsive neurosis)
4. Post-traumatic stress disorder
5. Atypical anxiety disorder

Without listing all the technical criteria required for an official *DSM-III* diagnosis, perhaps a summary highlighting the differences among these disorders will be important for understanding the models presented in this chapter.

Phobic Disorders

Phobias are persistent and irrational fears that result in avoidance behaviors. Examples include fear of open places, social situations, heights, closed spaces, certain animals, etc. Phobic individuals will increasingly constrict their normal activities as a result of the phobias, until the fears or avoidance behaviors dominate their life.

Anxiety States

This category has two major subdivisions. The first is made up of acute panic attacks which are characterized by a combination of dyspnea, palpitations, chest pain or discomfort, choking or smothering sensations, dizziness, vertigo or unsteady feelings, feelings of unreality, paresthesias, hot and cold flashes, sweating, faintness, trembling or shaking, and the fear of dying, going crazy, or doing something uncontrolled during an attack. The precipitant may or may not be apparent.

The second is a form of anxiety which is more generalized and persistent. It may consist of signs of motor tension (shakiness, jitteriness, jumpiness, trembling, tension, muscle aches, fatigability, inability to relax, eyelid twitch, furrowed brow, strained face, fidgeting, restlessness, easy startle); signs of autonomic hyperactivity (sweating, heart pounding or racing, cold and clammy hands, dry mouth, dizziness, light-headedness, paresthesias, upset stomach, hot or cold spells, frequent urination, diarrhea, discomfort in the pit of the stomach, lump in the throat, flushing, pallor, high resting pulse and respiration rate); apprehensive expectation (anxiety, worry, fear, rumination, and anticipation of misfortune to self or others); vigilance and scanning (hyperattentiveness resulting in distractibility, difficulty in concentrating, insomnia, feeling on edge, irritabiltiy, impatience).

Obsessive–Compulsive Disorder

Obsessions are recurrent, persistent ideas, thoughts, images, or impulses that are not experienced as voluntarily produced but rather as thoughts that invade consciousness and are experienced as senseless or repugnant. Attempts are made to ignore or suppress them.

Compulsions are repetitive behaviors performed according to certain rules or in a stereotyped fashion. The individual generally recognizes the senselessness of the behavior and does not derive pleasure from carrying out the activity although it provides a release of tension.

Post-Traumatic Stress Disorder

This disorder occurs following exposure to "a recognizable stressor that would evoke significant symptoms of distress in almost anyone" (*DSM-III*, 1980). There are a variety of symptoms that can occur following such exposure, but they do not necessarily constitute the disorder. The syndrome occurs in only a certain proportion of exposed persons and has by now been well described in the literature (Horowitz, 1976). It basically consists of such phenomena as recurrent and intrusive reexperiencing of the trauma as evidenced by recurrent thoughts, feelings, and/or dreams. There is often a diminution of interest in the external world and a variety of symptoms from the following list: hyperalertness or exaggerated startle response, sleep disturbance, guilt about surviving, memory impairment or trouble concentrating, avoidance of activities that arouse recollection of the traumatic event, intensification of symptoms by exposure to events that symbolize or resemble the traumatic event.

Atypical Anxiety Disorder

This is a diagnostic category used to describe the situation in which the individual appears to have an anxiety disorder but does not meet the criteria for inclusion in one of the above categories.

Other Conceptualizations of Anxiety

Lest the *DSM-III* descriptions of anxiety become too reified, we should remember that there are other ways to conceptualize anxiety which may be relevant to our consideration of the different approaches to animal modeling. This relates to the issue of anxiety as a symptom, as a signal, or as a syndrome. The term is often used imprecisely, and especially in the development of animal models, we need to maintain clarity about how the term is being used. This can be done by clear specification of any intended analogy between a human phenomenon and the animal phenomenon being studied. Nemiah (1974), in the *American Handbook of Psychiatry,* summarized these issues well. The work of Horowitz (1976) on the conceptualization of stress responses and anxiety is also a seminal contribution. More recently, a growing literature about the neurobiology of anxiety has led to rethinking of some of the clinical concepts. The following is an attempt to summarize and integrate some of these trends as background for the review of animal models of anxiety.

Concerning anxiety we may have recently been rediscovering the wheel. This is particularly true with regard to panic attacks, a syndrome that some writers think they have just discovered. Nemiah (1974) quotes from Robert Burton's *Anatomy of Melancholy:*

> Many lamentable effects . . . this fear causeth in men, as to be red, pale, tremble, sweat; it makes sudden cold and heat to come over all the body, palpitation of the heart, syncope, etc. It amazeth many men that are to speak or show themselves in public assemblies or before some great personages. (cited in Nemiah, 1974, p. 91) [What better description of panic attacks could one want?]

To understand current conceptualizations and controversies about anxiety, it is necessary to go back at least to the time of Janet. As Nemiah points out, the syndromes of hysteria and hypochondriasis had for centuries been considered as clinical entities. However, Janet was one of the first 20th-century psychiatrists to focus in an organized way on phobias, obsessions, and compulsions. In his classification there were two major categories: hysteria, which included all of the classical mental and sensorimotor dissociative phenomena, and psychasthenia, a mixture of all the other neurotic manifestations parceled out by modern diagnosticians among the various psychoneuroses.

Janet's work not withstanding, it is Freud's writing on anxiety that began a transition in our conceptualization of anxiety. Frued's earliest view was that anxiety was the mental state produced by toxic products of frustrated sexual libido. He later abandoned this conept, and in *Inhibi-*

tions, Symptoms, and Anxiety (Freud, 1961), he described anxiety as, like fear, a signal of approaching danger, a signal that mobilitzes the ego's defenses. The danger could be either external or internal. When the danger was external the signal was called fear, and when it was internal the signal was called anxiety. Anxiety thus signals internal danger. The internal danger comes from threatened breakthrough of ego-alien impulses that have been repressed. This was the earliest meaning of the "signal" function of anxiety. In this context anxiety was considered central for the theory of symptom formation in the etiology of neuroses. This concept of the central role of anxiety in psychological functioning was accepted by psychoanalysts, and anxiety itself was generally recognized by psychiatrists as a neurotic symptom.

Freud, however, also suggested that anxiety belonged to a specific diagnostic entity and that there was a specific syndrome called "anxiety neurosis." He described the symptoms of this syndrome as both chronic and acute. The two forms corresponding very closely to the *DSM-III* category of anxiety neurosis or anxiety states that were described at the beginning of this chapter.

Nemiah quotes from Freud's *Inhibitions, Symptoms, and Anxiety:*

> Anxiety attacks of this sort may consist of the feeling of anxiety alone, without any associated idea, or accompanied by the interpretation that is nearest to hand, such as ideas of the extinction of life or of a threat of madness; . . . or, finally, the feeling of anxiety may have linked to it a disturbance of one or more of the bodily functions such as respiration, heart action, vasomotor innervation of glandular activity. From this combination the patient picks out in particular now one, now another, factor. He complains of "spasms of the heart," "difficulty in breathing," "outbreaks of sweating," "ravenous hunger," and such like; and, in his description, the feeling of anxiety often recedes into the background or is referred to quite unrecognizably as "being unwell," feeling uncomfortable, and so on. (1974, p. 93)

The concept of anxiety as playing a central role in psychic functioning was readily accepted into mainstream psychoanalysis. This mainly involved an understanding of anxiety as a symptom. However, the syndrome of anxiety neurosis, suggested by Freud, was not accepted until much later, indeed not until after World War II. We have now rediscovered it, and it has found its way into the new nomenclature.

To summarize, anxiety can be either a symptom or a specific syndrome. In the development of animal models for anxiety it is important to be clear how one is using the term. The literature is very confusing in this regard. As a symptom, anxiety is closely related to a wide variety of mental disorders such as phobias, obsessive–compulsive neuroses, depression, etc. As a specific syndrome, anxiety neurosis has certain hallmark features and is characteristically unrelated to any specific event or reason. In the development of models it is important to remember that most forms of the anxiety neurosis syndrome are seemingly unrelated to any specific inducing condition, although it is generally thought that developmental factors play an important role. It will be apparent that none of the model systems reviewed model the syndrome of anxiety neurosis. Virtually all come closer to modeling fear or learning in an acute form.

Of vital importance in the development of any animal model is the assessment of behavior. This is no less true in the case of anxiety. Since we cannot talk to animals, what are the defining characteristics of human anxiety (symptom or syndrome) that we should be attempting to measure in animals? The following is a list of some phenomena typical of anxiety in humans. It is being given for reference, so that as the discussion of model systems is developed, judgments can be formed about how well the models measure up to the criteria of behavioral similarity. Since the inducing conditions for many forms of human anxiety are unknown, it is impossible to use induction as a criterion. This leaves the criteria of behavioral similarity, of treatment responsiveness, and of mechanisms. But not enough is known about the mechanisms of anxiety to use this as a criterion either. Therefore, we are left with behavioral similarities and treatment responsiveness criteria. Some of the phenomena of classic anxiety include the following:

1. Somatic
   a. tachycardia
   b. increased blood pressure
   c. flushing
   d. sweating
   e. increased muscular tension
   f. diarrhea
   g. palpitations
   h. hyperventilation
   i. dizziness
2. Experiential
   a. feelings of dread
   b. panic feelings
   c. confusion
   d. inability to concentrate
   e. feeling tense, on edge, irritable
   f. worry, fear, rumination
   g. hyperattentiveness resulting in distractibility

Animal Models of Anxiety

Operant Conditioning Paradigms

The basic strategy behind these models is to use operant techniques to elicit a behavior with a high frequency of occurrence. After the response is well established, the behavior is then suppressed by punishing it when it occurs. The analogy to fear is the conditioned association between the behavior and the punishment. Potential antianxiety drugs are screened by their ability to restore responding to its presuppression levels (Cook and Davidson, 1973; Cook and Sepinwall, 1975a,b; Davidson and Cook, 1969; Hill and Tedeschi, 1971; McMillan, 1975).

One of the best known of such tests is the Geller Conflict Test (Geller and Seifter, 1960; Geller, Kulak, and Seifter, 1962; Howard and Pollard, 1977). It is widely used in screening for potential antianxiety drugs. In the original Geller paradigm, rats were trained on a multiple variable interval 2-minute/CRF schedule for milk reinforcement. This means there was a two-component operant behavior schedule. In the variable interval (VI) portion, signalled by one stimulus, bar pressing is reinforced at variable intervals with the mean interval being 2 minutes. In the continuous reinforcement (CRF) portion, signalled by a different stimulus, every bar pressing is reinforced. When footshock is given concurrently with the positive reinforcement, response rates are suppressed. Drug-induced increases in the rate of punished responding are interpreted as an index of antianxiety activity, whereas decreases in unpunished responding are interprated as indicating depressant activity. The type of behavior that originally had a high frequency of occurrence but was subsequently suppressed by certain manipulations is highly sensitive to the benzodiazepines and to meprobamate, but not chlorpromazine. In general, this test, along with many subsequent modifications, identifies clinically active anxiolytic agents, predicts their clinical potency, and is generally insensitive to stimulant, antipsychotic, antidepressant, or analgesic drugs. It seems to work in different species and to be relatively independent of the schedules of positive reinforcement or punishment. Thus, this operant conflict approach has high empirical validity in terms of predicting clinical drug responsiveness.

This model, involving conflict behavior, has been used more recently to evaluate several biochemical hypotheses concerning the mechanism of action for the antianxiety, or what is termed the "emotional analgesic," properties of benzodiazepines. With the increasing interest in the possible neurobiological substrates of anxiety, the availability of a paradigm in which the mechanism of drug action can be explored simultaneously with measures of operant behavior is necessary for future research in this area (Lippa, Greenblatt, and Pelham, 1977). Over the last few years, with the identification of benzodiazepine receptor sites, evidence has begun to accumulate that these receptors may mediate the therapeutic effects of such drugs. The relationship of these receptor sites for benzodiazepines to our understanding of the neurobiological mechanisms of anxiety states is complex and remains an active and exciting area of investigation. The involvement of various neurotransmitter systems with these receptor sites is important to understand, and the continuing development of experimental systems in which these complex interrelationships can be studied would be helpful. There are a number of theories, especially relating the GABA and/or the serotonin systems to the effects of the anxiolytic drugs. However, there are many different components of anxiety, and different neurotransmitters may be involved with each. For example, the muscle relaxant or anticonvulsant properties may be neurochemically mediated in one way, but the anxiolytic effects as revealed in conflict paradigms may be mediated by other neurotransmitters. It is increasingly important to have careful behavioral descriptions along with the increasingly specific neurochemical technology.

How well do response-contingent punishment paradigms in animals model human anxiety from other standpoints? Howard and others (Cook and Sepinwall, 1975a,b; Fischman, Schuster, and Uhlenhuth, 1977; Howard and Pollard, 1977) have written about this relationship, but there is not a large literature. The suppression of responding in the punishment paradigms has been considered as a passive avoidance response, and it has been suggested that a component of the human anxiety in psychoneurotic states arises from passive avoidance of social situations. This is a complex area in human anxiety. Some would interpret human avoidance of social situations in other ways, but this debate may not be directly relevant to animal studies. The connection between response-contingent paradigms in animals and human anxiety has been taken one step further. The response suppression produced by punishment in these tests has been related to the response suppression produced by punishment of appropriate responses in childhood which, in turn, can lead to anxiety in later life. These possible connections are, of course, highly speculative but do indicate that these paradigms can be related on a theoretical level to human clinical theories. The problem in evaluating this theory is that specific etiologies for human anxiety are lacking.

As far as other similarities go, visual monitoring of the animals in a conflict situation reveals many unusual behaviors which have been likened to those in anxious humans. There are "abortive bar presses, discontinuous or jerky movements, and other bizarre behaviors." These are reported to return to normal with treatment with anxiolytics. Perhaps of most interest in making comparisons with humans is the fact that humans have indeed been run in experimental conflict paradigms and have been reported to show behaviors similar to those shown by animals.

In summary, the effect of anxiolytics is to attenuate the suppressive effects of punishment on responding. Perhaps this happens by reversing passive avoidance behavior. Procedures that use active avoidance responses have not found any specific effects of the anxiolytics. Said another way, the anxiolytics are disinhibiting behavior in this paradigm, and there is a literature which supports this as a possible mechanism by which the anxiolytics work. Given the advancements in the neurobiology of anxiety and the identification of benzodiazepine receptors, interesting connections which involve behavior, drugs, and neurobiology can now be pondered. It is important to remember, however, that the major reason for developing such tests was for empirical drug screening, not for studying the mechanisms of anxiety. Behavioral paradigms created for other reasons can, however, have great mechanistic spin-offs if neurobiological determinists do not push them too early and too far in ways that make sophisticated behavioral assessments impossible.

A number of additional variables of punished responding have been studied. These include the drug history of the animal, the dose of the drug administered, the type of stimulus used to punish responding, the intensity and duration of the punishing stimulus, the control rate and pattern of punished responding, the schedule of positive reinforcement maintaining the punished responding, the species of animal, the deprivation state of the animal, the behavioral history of the animal, and the nature of the required response. It is not known how all of these variables influence the effects of drugs on punished responding, only that many of them do.

In general, it is true that drugs used clinically as minor tranquilizers increase rates of punished responding, as do the barbiturates, but that nonbarbiturate sedative hypnotics, major tranquilizers, and amphetamines do not. However, there are a number of exceptions. Under the right conditions, amphetamines, morphine, and chlorpromazine can all increase rates of responding suppressed by punishment, and when punishment does not markedly suppress responding, minor tranquilizers and barbiturates do not increase rates of punished responding. However, the test if run properly is reasonably specific (Cook and Davidson, 1975; Cook and Sepinwall, 1975a,b; McMillan, 1975).

A modification of the Geller Conflict Test, developed by Cook and Davidson (1973), consists of a multiple schedule of reinforcement in which the alternating components are a variable interval 30-second (VI 30) schedule reinforced by food in the presence of a white houselight, and a fixed ratio 10-response (FR 10) schedule reinforced simultaneously with food and footshock in the presence of a red houselight. The development of suppression after shock was introduced during the FR components. As the shock intensity was gradually increased, the FR response rates, which were initially higher than the VI rates, decreased to approximately 10% of their original values. At the same time there was an increase in unpunished VI rates, (i.e., a contrast effect). The suppressed FR rates were operationally designated as conflict behavior. Psychotropic drugs were studied for their ability to attenuate the conflict by increasing responding during the punishment periods. Increases in responding during the punishment periods were produced by benzodiazepines, carbamic acid esters, and some barbiturates. This did not appear to be due to any general stimulation, since amphetamine actually produced a greater amount of suppression during FR segments. Inactive compounds included neuroleptics, antidepressants, antihistamines, and morphine.

A Model Based on Alteration of Locus Coeruleus Function

Another proposed animal model of anxiety is based on studies of the locus coeruleus (Huang, Redmond, Snyder, and Maas, 1975; Redmond, 1977, 1979, 1983; Redmond, Huang, Snyder, Maas, and Baulu, 1977).

The locus coeruleus is a brain structure which has a very high density of norepinephrine-containing neurons plus numerous projections to other brain regions. Various techniques to alter its function provide one way to learn more about the function of one noradrenergic system in brain. The system has been studied in the cat, macaque, and squirrel monkey. Techniques employed include electrical stimulation, ablation, and pharmacological probes. The details of these studies are too numerous for one chapter, but to summarize, the locus coeruleus has been studied in many species with variable results. There are significant species differences in the catecholamine-containing cells in the brain stem in addition to significant variations in behaviors. Cross-species reasoning from such studies is difficult, but a recent set of studies in nonhuman primates may be particularly relevant to animal models of anxiety.

Research groups studying the locus coeruleus have particularly measured behaviors associated with threats in monkeys. Their list of categories is derived from field investigations in which such behaviors have been noted in situations of impending aggression, danger, conflict, or uncertainty. They were then assessed in the laboratory in chair-restrained monkeys whose locus coeruleus functions had been altered in one way or another. Behavioral assessments were made from videotapes of the chaired monkeys which were housed in sound-dampened cubicles. The behavioral categories scored (Redmond, 1977) are listed so they can be compared with the previous listing of the phenomena of anxiety:

jump/startle	head turn
scratch	body shake
handwring	grind teeth
hair/skin pull	eat
self-mouth	drink
tongue movement	pout face/grunt purr
chew	lipsmack
grasp	grimace
clutch	threat
struggle	manipulate object
yawn	penile erection
freeze	defecate
self-groom	urinate
eye scan	vocalize
attend/scare	arm drop
lookout	sit quietly
brows up	drowsy
open mouth/brows up	eyes closed

Increasing locus coeruleus function, either by electrical stimulation or with drugs, led to an increase in threat-associated behaviors, whereas decreasing locus coeruleus function decreased threat-associated behaviors. Some have argued that "these behavioral effects are consistent with an essential role for the locus coeruleus in mediating anxiety and fear, and can be confirmed to some extent from human reports of the effects of some of these drugs and procedures" (Redmond, 1977, p. 297).

The following three criteria for a central neurophysiological model of anxiety have been presented, and data is discussed in this context.

The first criterion is that there should be quantifiable objective behavioral measures which meet the following conditions:

1. They are produced by the conditions which produce the emotion in humans.
2. They are quantitatively increased with increasing intensity of fear or anxiety producing stimuli.
3. They are selectively dininished, after identical stimuli, by pharmacologic agents which are anxiolytic in humans.
4. They correlate with the other peripheral and central manifestations of anxiety or fear in humans (pulse rate, tremor, skin conductance changes, cortisol secretion, etc).

It has been argued that the behavioral measures associated with locus coeruleus function in primates are the same ones that change with environmental stimuli associated with fear in humans and that they are lessened by diazepam. However, it has also been pointed out that this approach does not permit a distinction between fear as a response to an externally threatening situation and anxiety, which is typically more free floating and less related to a specific environment precipitant. This is a problem with much of the animal modeling of anxiety literature in which the terms *anxiety, fear,* and *learning* are often used interchangeably.

The second criterion is that the behavioral and physiological changes should be reproduced by alterations in central physiological function. These are the mechanisms criteria:

1. The central systems altered should be anatomically and neurochemically connected to other areas and systems known to regulate physiological manifestations or correlates of anxiety. What are these areas in the case of human anxiety? Too little is known to use this as a validating criterion.

2. Low-intensity electrical stimulation should produce or increase the behavioral and physiological manifestations and approximate qualitatively and quantitatively those resulting from fear-producing nonpainful stimuli.

3. Specific electrolytic lesions should diminish or abolish the behavioral and physiological manifestations in response to environmental stimuli effective in producing them in normal animals.

4. Specific biochemical alterations in the function of the same areas should have effects consistent with the functional effects of low-inten-

sity electrical stimulation of the areas or lesions of the areas. Ideally, these same agents should also be anxiolytic or produce anxiety in humans.

Using this set of criteria, a speculative anatomy of locus–coeruleus-mediated anxiety is presented. It is proposed that the effects of alteration of locus coeruleus or dorsal bundle activity are similar to those seen after exposure to fear-producing stimuli.

The third criterion is that the central correlates of function in the proposed relevant areas or systems should exist based on the following:

1. Evidence of decreased function for all agents which are anxiolytic in humans

2. Evidence of increased function for all procedures, stimuli, or drugs which increase or produce anxiety or fear in humans

3. Peripheral evidence of function as available from humans not inconsistent with the proposed central function

Those supporting this theory review a variety of psychopharmacological literature which they feel supports the first two conditions and some human research of the amine system in fearful or anxious humans.

Their general conclusion is that based on the data so far available, the locus coeruleus is essential, though not sufficient, for the behavioral and physiological expression of anxiety. Other areas are required. The locus coeruleus is likened to "an alarm system."

Throughout the discussion of this particular approach to modeling, the terms *fear* and *anxiety* are used interchangeably. The relationship between these two states are complex. What is being described are fear-produced behavioral changes that can be produced behaviorally and by manipulation of the locus coeruleus. These results may model, on some level, acute fear, but study of this state may or may not tell us anything about the origins of human anxiety. This does not mean the approach is not useful. It is, especially in studying the relationships between central noradrenergic functioning and a specified set of behaviors. The debate centers about to what extent these behaviors are phenomenologically similar to those seen in clinical anxiety. However, such debates should not cloud the significance of this line of research in clarifying the relationship between alteration in the functioning of a given brain region and behaviors shown by different species of animals. As previously stated, it is not necessary to anchor a given line of research to a specific clinical syndrome, and this principle is illustrated again with the locus coeruleus work.

A Model Based on Studies of Aplysia

Kandel has proposed that not only anxiety as a general state, but several specific subcategories of anxiety, can be modeled in the sea snail, *Aplysia*. Because of its relatively simple nervous system, it is contended that the molecular basis of anxiety can be studied in this type of animal preparation. There is currently great interest in this approach because it offers the advantage of more direct approaches to studying the cellular mechanisms of behavior. "Behavior" in this type of preparation has a very different meaning from that in some of the previous models. It is not social behavior and is closest to a variant of conditioning paradigms that have been utilized for some time in the animal modeling field.

First, some clarification of Kandel's use of the word *anxiety* is needed. He basically uses Klein's proposed subdivision of anxiety, which itself derives from earlier conceptualizations of anxiety by Freud and others. According to this scheme there are two forms of anxiety—anticipatory, or signaled, anxiety and chronic anxiety (Kandel, 1983). (There is actually a third form called panic attacks, but most of this chapter focuses on anticipatory and chronic anxiety.)

As described by Freud, anticipatory, or signaled, anxiety is an acquired fear response in anticipation of a real external danger. Freud distinguished this from actual or automatic anxiety which is an inborn response (rather than acquired) to external or internal danger. The point is that anticipatory anxiety is acquired and is triggered by a cue that has come to be associated with danger.

Chronic anxiety, by contrast, is a persistent feeling of tension that cannot be related to any obvious external source. It probably has its origins in the process of development and needs to be understood from a combination of psychodynamic, physiological, cognitive, and neurobiological frameworks.

Kandel argues that, in *Aplysia*, classically conditioned fear models anticipatory anxiety, and what is termed "long-term sensitization" models chronic anxiety. The basic paradigm used is as follows. The aversive or unconditioned stimulus (US) is strong shock to the head of *Aplysia*. This is followed by the trauma of a weak test probe to the tail, which elicits an unconditioned reflex or instinctive response—in the case of *Aplysia*, escape locomotion and other defensive reflexes. A conditioned stimulus (CS) does not elicit the reflex response before repeated pairing with the unconditioned stimulus. In the case of *Aplysia* the conditioned stimulus is extract of shrimp. By pairing with the US (head shock), the CS (extract of shrimp) can come to elicit the reflex or unconditioned response. This is fairly straightforward classical or Pavlovian conditioning, which is reviewed in the historical chapter and has been used for some time in the study of experimental neuroses. Thus, the behavioral aspects of this particular experimental system are not new. However, some newer and important neurophysiological techniques have been applied in the study of these paradigms, and some reconceptualization of their relationship to clinical anxiety has occurred.

Many workers have speculated about the relationship of aversive conditioning paradigms in animals to human anxiety. On the one hand, there is the situation where the CS serves as a cue predicting the occurrence of the US and various behavioral changes occur, presumably in anticipation of the US. This has been likened by a number of investigators to anticipatory or signaled anxiety. This is illustrated in the sea snail work where exposure to the extract of shrimp alone comes to elicit the withdrawal and reflex responses. The term chronic anxiety or long-term sensitization has been widely used to describe the state in which there is repeated exposure to the US alone, without any cueing or prior exposure to the CS. Seligman and others have speculated about the role of unpredictability or uncontrollability as a factor in mediating this response.

Kandel uses "anxiety" to describe the withdrawal reflexes produced in *Aplysia*. Similar terms have been used by earlier workers to describe unconditioned or conditioned responses in other kinds of animals. The work with *Aplysia* is new, as is the neurophysiological work to be described. However, it is not appropriate to use the word *anxiety* to describe the changes in *Aplysia* in the same way the word is used to refer to subjectively experienced states of mind in humans. There is no argument with this being a kind of learning and providing an experimental system in which the cellular basis of this learning can be studied. Indeed, Kandel himself makes clear that the mechanisms of anxiety in simple animals are not likely to be identical to that in humans, but that regardless of this it is important to discover the mechanisms of how animals learn about threatening stimulus configurations. I would agree that this is where the major contributions of this line of work have been made.

In a classic series of neurophysiological experiments the neural circuits involved with the gill withdrawal reflex of *Aplysia* during sensitization-exposure to the US without prior cueing by an CS have been studied (Bailey and Chen, 1983; Bailey, Hawkins, Chen, and Kandel, 1981; Brunnel, Castellucci, and Kandel, 1976; Castellucci, Pinsker, Kupferman, and Kandel, 1970; Castellucci, Kandel, Schwartz, Wilson, Nairn, and Greengard, 1980; Castellucci, Nairn, Greengard, Schwartz, and Kandel, 1982; Hawkins, Castellucci, and Kandel, 1981; Kandel, 1976;

Kandel and Schwartz, 1982; Klein and Kandel, 1980; Siegelbaum, Camardo, and Kandel, 1982; Walters, Carew, and Kandel, 1979, 1981).

Remember that this kind of learning has been explicitly proposed as a model for "chronic anxiety." Researchers have reported that this type of exposure leads to an enhancement of the connections made by the sensory neurons on their target cells (presynaptic facilitation). Serotonin is the neurotransmitter used by these facilitation cells which act as a defensive arousal system. Serotonin, in turn, causes an increase in intracellular messenger cyclic AMP in sensory neurons, which in turn facilitates transmitter release from the terminals of sensory neurons. Cyclic AMP activates a protein kinase, and kinase activation leads to closing of a certain kind of potassium channel and an increased influx of calcium. To quote Kandel:

> Thus, we have been able to take the analysis of a form of anxiety from the behavior of the intact animal to the neural circuit of the behavior and to some of the critical cells involved. Within these critical cells (the sensory neurons of the reflex) we localized the change to a particular component of the neuron, the presynaptic terminals, and demonstrated that the expression of anxiety involves enhancememnt of transmitter release. We found that the molecular mechanism of this enhancement is protein phosphorylation, which leads to a broadening of the action potential and a greater influx of calcium. We are now able to focus on the individual protein molecules modulated by learning and explore them in a behavioral as well as a biochemical context. (1983, p. 1,286)

Some would prefer to substitute "protective behavior" for anxiety in the above quote. In addition to the above changes, morphological changes have been reported in sensitized animals. Studies compared sensory neurons from chronically sensitized animals and control animals and found that the active zones, which are where the vesicles are loaded onto release sites from which they subsequently discharge their contents, were increased in number and in size.

This line of reasoning, after offering a molecular explanation for what these researchers call chronic anxiety, raises the possibility that anxiety might involve alterations in gene expression based on the power of experience in modifying brain function through altering synaptic strength. This is not a new concept, and the details of it are not appropriate for this chapter. Such a possible mechanism exists for all forms of psychopathology, not just anxiety. What is of considerable relevance is the assertion that, in contrast to anxiety being a result of alterations of gene expression, schizophrenia and depression involve alteration in gene structure. Based on this speculation the view is that these illnesses do not involve exaggeration of normal adaptive processes and therefore are characteristic human illnesses. Since fear or anxiety is a general adaptive mechanism found in simple as well as complex animals, it can be studied in animal models. This line of reasoning is flawed in several respects. Even though schizophrenia and depression clearly have genetic components and could conceivably involve actual alterations in gene structure (though such evidence is not yet available), they nevertheless might have a significant interaction with developmental and environmental variables. There are few diseases involving alteration of the structure of genes in which this alone is sufficient to explain the occurence of the illness. Furthermore, even if schizophrenia did not involve normal adaptive processes gone awry, this does not mean that they cannot be studied in animal models. Arteriosclerosis is not a normal adaptive process, and yet it has been usefully studied in animal models. There is no inherent reason why aspects of schizophrenia cannot usefully be studied in animal models as well as anxiety can. There should be little doubt from work done by many individuals that experience is a powerful influence on neurobiological functioning and that virtually all diseases involve complex interactions among genetic, developmental, and social variables.

Models Based Primarily on Social Manipulations

It is in this area that one encounters terms such as *fear, anxiety, agitation, stress,* and *neurosis* being used interchangeably, with a resultant extreme degree of confusion. For example, the initial stage of reaction to separation has historically been labeled the agitation, or protest, stage. More recently it has been conceptualized by some in an anxiety context (Suomi, Kraemer, Baysinger, and Delizio, 1981). The first phase of reaction to separation in rhesus monkeys is characterized, as previously discussed, by hyperactivity. It has also been found that the infants have marked activation of the pituitary–adrenal system and an increase in the enzymes involved in catecholamine synthesis (Breese, Smith, Mueller, Howard, Prange, Lipton, Young, McKinney, and Lewis, 1973). These findings and others, which support the view of separation as a very powerful event from both behavioral and neurobiological standpoints, are consistent with a large body of literature regarding the behavioral and biological effects of a variety of stressors. It is not yet known to what extent this initial stage of reaction responds to anxiolytic pharmacological agents and how specific this response may be. This would be an important line of research to pursue. It is interesting to speculate about the ability of such stressors to induce benzodiazepine receptor sites in brain. It is known, for example, that selection of emotionality in at least one rat strain is associated with the number of benzodiazepine receptor sites in brain. In general, the initial agitation, or protest, stage in reaction to separation has been far less studied than the subsequent despair, or depression, stage. One of the interesting facts is that the protest stage is nearly universal, whereas the despair stage is much more variable.

The initial protest stage following maternal separation has even been likened to a panic attack, and the fact that monkeys on imipramine do not exhibit either the protest or despair stage has been used as support for this argument (Suomi et al., 1978, 1981). However, in the imipramine study the medication was begun during the depressive phase and continued throughout subsequent separations. It affected the behavior in both stages, and it is impossible, from that study, to determine which was primary and which was secondary. What is needed is a series of pharmacological trials with antianxiety drugs, with antidepresants, and with neuropleptics.

Other experimental situations in primates which have been reported to model anxiety include introduction of strangers, rearing in conditions of social deprivation followed by exposure to a more socially stimulating environment, and early experience with a rejecting real or surrogate mother. There is one report to suggest that early autonomic responsivity, as measured by heart rate change in response to certain stimuli, correlates with later responses to certain stressors, but this needs to be replicated (Suomi et al., 1981).

Phobias and Other Neuroses

This area has recently been well reviewed in an article by Isaac Marks (1977). First, Marks reminds us of the distinction between *fear*, which comes from an Old English word for sudden calamity or danger, and *anxious*, which is from the Greek root meaning "press tight" or "strangle." According to Marks and others, fear is an emotion produced by present or impending danger; the cause is apparent. Anxiety, on the other hand, is the emotion produced when the cause is vague or less understandable. Fear can lead to either freezing or becoming mute. Much stress literature reports these behaviors (e.g., rats freezing in an open field) as being stress.

There has been one study which had potential for stimulating further work on phobias, but as yet no one has followed through. In this study, monkeys in social isolation were shown slides on the inside of their cages. They also had levers they could press to make the pictures appear. None of the pictures disturbed them except those of other monkeys threatening, especially when the isolated monkeys were about 2½ to 4 months of age. Marks suggests that there may be innate mechanisms of recognition in monkeys that lead to social interaction and learned modification of the innate reaction. The speculation is that during this time of 2½ to 4 months, monkeys may be particularly prone to acquire new fears of neutral stimuli that are paired with innately fear-releasing stimuli like threat. It is surprising that very few proposed models of anxiety incorporate developmental considerations, in view of the extensive clinical literature about the developmental origins of anxiety (Sackett, 1966).

Marks discusses conditioning models and theories in relation to anxiety and phobia models and points to a number of their shortcomings in relation to human phobias. There are many animal experiments that assume conditioned fear as well as avoidance conditioned by trauma that are models of human phobic (or anxiety) reactions. Several of these have been discussed in this chapter. While it is true that such induction techniques do produce fear of relatively specific stimuli and enable the study of variables that are important for the learning of fear in humans, a clearly definable event (i.e., a definable US) can rarely be found at the start of human phobias (or anxiety).

Marks thinks that research on animals has little to tell us about human anxieties that exist internally and symbolically, often without observable motor or autonomic concomitants. The operational definition of anxiety is difficult, and Marks feels that Pavlovian and Skinnerian conditioning paradigms are useless for modeling human phobias (anxieties). Human phobias and anxiety just do not fit into conditioning language or paradigms. He feels that conditioning language makes assumptions about etiology and treatment that are not borne out in practice, and that the terminology is difficult to apply to clinical events.

One other approach to the study of phobias has been done. This involves the development of two lines of pointer dogs (Dykman and Gantt, 1960; Dykman, Gantt, and Whitehorn, 1956; Dykman, Murphree, and Ackerman, 1966; Dykman, Murphree, and Peters, 1969; Dykman, Murphree, and Reese, 1979; Murphree, 1974; Murphree and Dykman, 1965; Murphree and Newton, 1971; Murphree, Deluca, and Angel, 1974; Newton, Murphree, and Dykman, 1970; Newton, Chapin, and Murphree, 1976; Newton, Dykman, and Chapin, 1978; Peters, 1966; Peters, Murphree, and Dykman, 1967; Walk, Murphree, and Angel, 1976).

One line was bred for fearfulness and lack of friendliness toward people. Another was bred for the opposite characteristics. The basic hypothesis of this work was that inheritance would determine in large part many behavioral characteristics of the dogs, including susceptibility to breakdown under acute and chronic stress. Throughout 10 generations, about 80% of each litter were similar in temperament to the parents. Through this process of selection and inbreeding, it was possible to establish the two lines of dogs and to study their behavior on a number of parameters. The "phobic" line was extremely timid, avoided humans, and showed decreased exploratory activity. These dogs showed an excessive startle response, a slower heart rate, and an increased incidence of atrioventricular heart block. Interestingly, even those with the most severe disturbance could learn operant conditioning bar pressing, but it was necessary to facilitate this process with benzodiazepines—the most efficacious drugs. Amphetamine and cocaine disrupted the behavioral responses of genetically nervous dogs to a far greater extent than they did to the stable line (Angel, Murphree, and Deluca, 1974).

Could these pointer dogs genetically predisposed to nervous behavior be rehabilitated? By means of a program of gradual desensitization involving graduated exposure, reciprocally competitive responses, and social facilitation, it was possible to train them as hunting dogs. However, this rehabilitated behavior did not extend to laboratory tests (McBryde and Murphree, 1974; Murphree, Angel, and Deluca, 1974).

This same group also reported biochemical data to suggest hyperresponsiveness of the central nervous system noradrenergic and cholinergic systems along with a hyporesponsiveness of the serotonergic system related to the genetically expressed aberrant behavior (Angel, Deluca, and Murphree, 1976; Deluca, Murphree, and Angel, 1974).

A number of clinically important questions are raised by this work with dogs. One is whether the inheritance factor, even in human phobics, might be greater than present techniques can measure. Another is the interaction between a genetic predisposition and developmental experiences and subsequent neurobiology. It is true that with dogs we are unlikely to unravel molecular mechanisms of this altered behavior, but the work on other levels is extremely important.

General Discussion and Conclusions

The following conclusions can be drawn from a review of proposed animal models of anxiety:

1. Anxiety is a human state that is poorly defined from an operational or phenomenological standpoint. Many of the core defining characteristics of human anxiety are experiential and psychophysiological. Therefore it is difficult to evaluate the animal models from the standpoint of behavioral similarities.

2. Acute agitation or fear, or what some might even call panic, can be reproduced in animals relatively easily. A variety of physical and psychological stressors can do this. The relationship of acute fear to the more usual anxiety states in humans, which are usually chronic, needs to be reconceptualized.

3. Certain types of conflict-induced suppression of responding paradigms have high empirical validity in terms of predicting clinical antianxiety drug responsiveness and deserve further study with regard to possible underlying neurobiological or behavioral mechanisms. Would animals which have had behavioral induction of suppressed responding have altered locus coeruleus functioning? These are important questions regarding the interface between social and neurobiological functioning.

   There is great potential in such paradigms for studies involving mechanisms of antianxiety drug action without any necessity to defend the model either in terms of behavioral similarity or etiology. However, in regard to the latter, these kinds of studies have been conceptually related to the etiology of human anxiety. These speculative considerations need to be further evaluated.

   Developmental factors have not been studied in relation to this approach but could be in the future. For example, what effect would alteration of social rearing conditions have on conflict-induced suppression of responding and on the effects of drugs in altering this.

   Likewise, the effects of social behavior outside the specific testing paradigm have not been evaluated, but they could be, especially in different species. This would be very interesting in relation to chronic anxiety.

4. Certain conditioning paradigms in a variety of vertebrates and invertebrates have value in their own right in studies of learning, but they are unconvincing as models of anxiety, for which they have been proposed. Mark's criticisms of such models will not be repeated here, but it is time we focus elsewhere in our search for experimental systems for the study of anxiety.

5. With regard to central nervous system models, especially locus coeruleus models, they have the enormous advantage of permitting the careful study of a specified set of behaviors in relation to

central manipulation of a given neurochemical system. It would be very important to relate this approach to the other models. For example, how would alteration of locus coeruleus function affect conflict-induced suppression of responding and vice versa.

6. It is critical that one be very careful with terminology. The terms *neurosis, fear, anxiety,* and *agitation* may not be describing the same thing. As a matter of fact, animal studies have the potential for helping with this semantic confusion.

7. Increasing attention to developmental factors in a number of animal species is important, given some of the etiological theories of the development of human anxiety states. Is it possible by altered social and/or neurobiological development to produce an animal preparation that reacts to social situations later in life in some altered fashion that we can measure? These kinds of paradigms, then, would permit mechanism as well as drug treatment studies.

Summary of Key Points

- *Most animal modeling work involves the study of animals reacting to external threats, conflicts, trauma, etc. In this context, fear and/or learning are probably being studied more than anxiety.*

- *The concepts of anxiety in general, and of animal models in particular, are being modified so as to be in a formative stage.*

- *The basic strategy behind the models being used most frequently involves the use of operant techniques to elicit a behavior with a high frequency of occurrence. After a response is well established, the behavior is then suppressed by punishment. Potential antianxiety drugs are screened by their ability to restore responding to its presuppression levels. This general approach has high empirical validity in terms of predicting clinical drug responsiveness and has more recently been used to begin investigations about the neurobiology of anxiety.*

- *The relationship of response-contingent punishment paradigms in animals to human anxiety is controversial. The suppression of responding in the punishment paradigms has been considered a passive avoidance response, and it has been suggested that a component of human anxiety can arise from passive avoidance of social situations. Others do not agree with this extension and would interpret human avoidance of social situations in other ways. Other theoretical extensions to human anxiety have been made from these kinds of animal studies.*

- *Another model is based on alteration of locus coeruleus function. The function is altered by electrical stimulation or by drugs, and the behavioral response studied. Some think that the behavioral effects are consistent with an essential role for the locus coeruleus in mediating anxiety and fear. Debate centers about to what extent these behaviors are phenomenologically similar to those seen in clinical anxiety and the relationship between fear behaviors and anxiety-type behaviors.*

- *An additional approach to anxiety has been suggested based on studies of the sea slug* Aplysia, *an invertebrate species. These studies are summarized, and the controversies surrounding the proposal that they represent an animal model of specific kinds of anxiety discussed.*

- *There are also models based primarily on social manipulations and those which emphasize developmental parameters. These approaches are newer, and the literature is not as large as in the other areas. Nevertheless, such approaches provide the potential for studying the interaction between developmental parameters, neurobiology, and drug responsiveness in relation to anxiety disorders.*

References

Angel, C. Murphree, O. D., and Deluca, D. C. (1974) The Effects of Chlordiazepoxide, Amphetamine, and Cocaine on Bar Press Behavior in Normal and Genetically Nervous Dogs *Diseases of the Nervous System* **35**:220–223.

Angel, C., Deluca, D. C., and Murphree, O. D. (1976) Probenecid Induced Accumulation of Cyclic Nucleotide, 5- Hydroxyindoleacetic Acid and Homovanillic Acid in Cisternal Spinal Fluid of Genetically Nervous Dogs. *Biological Psychiatry* **11**:753–763.

Bailey, C. H., and Chen, M. (1983) Morphological Basis of Long-Term Habituation and Sensitization in Aplysia *Science* **220**:91–93.

Bailey, C. H., Hawkins, R. D., Chen, M. C., and Kandel, E. R. (1981) Interneurons Involved in Mediation and Modulation of Gill-Withdrawal Reflex in Aplysia.IV. Morphological Basis of Presynaptic Facilitation. *Journal of Neurophysiology* **45**:340–360.

Breese, G., Smith, R. D., Mueller, R. A., Howard, J. L., Prange, A. J., Lipton, M. A., Young, L. D., McKinney, W. T., Lewis, J. K. (1973) Induction of Adrenal Catecholamine-Synthesizing Enzymes Following Mother–Infant Separation. *Nature: New Biology* **246**:94–96.

Brunelli, M., Castellucci, V., Kandel, E. R. (1976) Synaptic Facilitation and Behavioral Sensitization in Aplysia : Possible Role of Serotonin and Cyclic AMP. *Science* **194**:1178–1181.

Burton, R. (1964) *The Anatomy of Melancholy.* London: Dent.

Cannon, W. B. (1929) *Bodily Changes in Pain, Hunger, Fear, and Rage.* New York: D. Appleton and Company.

Castellucci, V., and Kandel, E. R. (1976) Presynaptic Facilitation As a Mechanism for Behavioral Sensitization in Aplysia. *Science* 194:1176–1178.

Castellucci, V., Pinsker, H., Kupferman, I., and Kandel, E. R. (1970) Neuronal Mechanisms of Habituation and Dishabituation of the Gill-Withdrawal Reflex in Aplysia. *Science* 167:1745–1748.

Castellucci, V. F., Kandel, E. R., Schwarz, J. H., Wilson, F. D., Nairn, A. C., and Greengard, P. (1980) Intracellular Injection of the Catalytic Subunit of Cyclic AMP-Dependent Protein Kinase Simulates Facilitation of Transmitter Release Underlying Behavioral Sensitization in Aplysia *Proceedings of the National Academy of Sciences* 77:7492–7496.

Castellucci, V. F., Nairn, A., Greengard, P., Schwarz, J. H., and Kandel, E. R. (1982) Inhibition of Adenosine 3'5'- Monophosphate Dependent Protein Kinase Blocks Presynaptic Facilitation in Aplysia *Journal of Neuroscience* 2:1673–1681.

Cook, L., and Davidson, A. B. (1973) Effects of Behaviorally Active Drugs in a Conflict–Punishment Procedure in Rats. In *The Benzodiazepines*, S. Garattini, E. Mussini, and L. O. Randall, (Eds.). New York: Raven Press.

Cook, L. and Sepinwall, J. (1975) Behavioral Analysis of the Effects and Mechanisms of Action of Benzodiazepines. In *Mechanism of Action of Benzodiazepines*, E. Costa, and P. Greengard (Eds.). New York: Raven Press.

Cook, L. and Sepinwall, J. (1975) Reinforcement Schedules and Extrapolations to Humans From Animals in Behavioral Pharmacology. *Federation Proceedings* 34:1889–1897.

Davidson, A. B., and Cook, L. (1969) Effects of Combined Treatment With Trifluoperazine HCL and Amobarbital on Punished Behavior in Rats. *Psychopharmacology* 15:159–168.

Deluca, D. C., Murphree, O. D., Angel, C. (1974) Biochemistry of Nervous Dogs *Pavlovian Journal of Biological Science* 9:136–148.

Diagnostic and Statistical Manual III (1980) Washington, D.C.: American Psychiatric Association.

Dykman, R. A., and Gantt, W. H. (1960) A Case of Experimental Neurosis and Recovery in Relation to the Orienting Response. *J. Psychol* 50:105–110.

Dykman, R. A., Gantt, W. H., and Whitehorm, J. C. (1956) Conditioning As Emotional Sensitization and Differentiation *Psychological Monographs* 70:1–17.

Dykman, R. A., Murphree, O. D., and Ackerman, P. T. (1966) Litter Patterns in the Offspring of Nervous and Stable Dogs: II. Autonomic and Motor Conditioning. *Journal of Nervous and Mental Diseases* 141:419–431.

Dykman, R. A., Murphree, O. D., and Peters, J. E. (1969) Like Begets Like. *Ann NY Acad Sci* 159:976–1007.

Dykman, R. A., Murphree, O. D., Reese, W. G. (1979) Familital Anthrophobia in Pointer Dogs. *Archives of General Psychiatry* 36:988–993.

Fischman, M., Schuster, C. R., and Uhlenhuth, E. H. (1977) Extension of Animal Models to Clincal Evaluation of Antianxiety Agents. In *Animal Models in Psychiatry and Neurology*, I. Hanin and E. Usdin (Eds.). New York: Pergamon Press.

Freud, S. (1961) *Inhibitions, Symptoms, and Anxiety*. In The Complete Psychological Works: Standard Edition (Vol. 20), J. Strachey (Ed. and trans.). London: Hogarth Press.

Geller, I., and Seifter, J. (1960) The Effects of Meprobamate, Barbiturates, *d*-Amphetamines and Promazine on Experimentally Induced Conflict in the Rat. *Psychopharmacologica* 1:482–492.

Geller, I., Kulak, J. T., and Seifter, J. (1962) The Effects of Chlordiazepoxide and Chlorpromazine on a Punishment Discrimination. *Psychopharmacologica* 3:374–385.

Hawkins, R. D., Castelluci, V. F., and Kandel, E. R. (1981) Interneruons Involved in

Mediation and Modulation of Gill-Withdrawal Reflex in Aplysia. II. Identified Neurons Produce Heterosynaptic Facilitation Contributing to Behavioral Sensitization. *Journal of Neurophysiology* **45:**315–339.

Hill, R. T., and Tedeschi, D. H. (1971) Animal Testing and Screening Procedures in Evaluating Psychotropic Drugs. In *An Introduction to Psychopharmacology*, R. Rech and K. Moore (Eds.). New York: Raven Press.

Horowitz, M. J. (1976) *Stress Response Syndromes.* New York: Jason Aronson, Inc..

Howard, J. L., and Pollard, G. T. (1977) The Geller Conflict Test: A Model of Anxiety and a Screening Procedure for Anxiolytics. In *Animal Models in Psychiatry and Neurology* I. Hanin and E. Usdin (Eds.). New York: Pergamon Press.

Huang, Y., Redmond, D. E., Snyder, D. R., and Maas, J. R. (1975) *In Vivo* Location and Destruction of the Locus Coeruleus in the Stumptail Macaque (*Macaca arcoides*). *Brain Research* **100:**157–162.

Kandel, E. R. (1976) *Cellular Basis of Behavior.* San Francisco: Freeman and Co.

Kandel, E. R. (1983) From Metapsychology to Molecular Biology: Explorations into the Nature of Anxiety. *American Journal of Psychiatry* **140:**1277–1993.

Kandel, E. R., and Schwarz, J. H. (1982) Molecular Biology of Learning: Modulation of Transmitter Release. *Science* **218:**433–443.

Klein, M. and Kandel, E. R. (1980) Mechanism of Calcium Current Modulation Underlying Presynaptic Facilitation and Behavioral Sensitization in Aplysia. *Proceedings of the National Academy of Sciences* **77:**6912–6916.

Lippa, A., Greenblatt, E. N., and Pelham, R. W. (1977) The Use of Animal Models for Delineating the Mechanisms of Action of Anxiolytic Agents. In *Animal Models in Psychiatry and Neurology* I. Hanin and E. Usdin (Eds.). New York: Pergamon Press.

Marks, I. (1977) Phobias and Obsessions: Clinical Phenomena in Search of a Laboratory Model. In *Psychopathology: Experimental Models*, J. Maser and M. Seligman (Eds.). San Francisco: Freeman.

McBryde, W. C., and Murphree, O. D. (1974) The Rehabilitation of Genetically Nervous dogs *Pavlov. J. Biol. Sci.* **9:**76–84.

McMillan, D. E. (1975) Determinants of Drug Effects on Punished Responding. *Federation Proceedings* **34:**1870–1879.

Murphree, O. D. (1974) Inheritance of Human Aversion and Inactivity in Two Strains of Pointer Dogs. *Biological Psychiatry* **7:**23–29.

Murphree, O. D., and Dykman, R. A. (1965) Litter Patterns in the Offspring of Nervous and Stable Dogs I: Behavioral Tests. *Journal of Nervous and Mental Diseases* **141:**321–332.

Murphree, O. D. and Newton, J. E. D. (1971) Crossbreeding and Special Handling of Genetically Nervous Dogs. *Pavlovian Journal of Biological Sciences* **6:**129–136.

Murphree, O. D., Angel, C., and Deluca, D. C. (1974) Limits of Therapeutic Change Specificity of Behavioral Modification in Genetically Nervous Dogs. *Biological Psychiatry* **9:**99–101.

Murphree, O. D., Deluca, D. C., and Angel, C. (1974) Psychopharmacologic Facilitation of Operant Conditioning of Genetically Nervous Catahoula and Pointer Dogs. *Pavlov J Biol Sci* **9:**17–24.

Nemiah, J. C. (1974) Anxiety: Signal, Symptom, and Syndrome. In *American Handbook of Psychiatry* Volume 3. New York: Basic Books.

Newton, J. E. D., Murphree, O. D., and Dykman, R. A. (1970) Sporadic Transient Atrioventricular Block and Slow Heart Rate in Nervous Pointer Dogs: A Genetic Study. *Pavlov J. Biol Sci* **5:**75–89.

Newton, J. E. D., Chapin, J. L. and Murphree, O. D. (1976) Correlations of Normality and

Nervousness With Cardiovascular Functions in Pointer Dogs. *Pavlovian Journal of Biological Sciences* 11:105–120.

Newton, J. E. D., Dykman, R. A., and Chapin, J. L. (1978) The Prediction of Abnormal Behavior from Autonomic Indices in Dogs. *Journal of Nervous and Mental Diseases* 66:6–16.

Peters, J. E. (1966) Typology of Dogs by the Conditional Reflex Method. *Pavlovian Journal of Biological Sciences* 1:235–250.

Peters, J. E., Murphree, O. D., Dykman, R. A. (1967) Genetically Determined Abnormal Behavior in Dogs: Some Implications for Psychiatry. *Pavlovian Journal of Biological Sciences* 2206–215.

Redmond, E. A. (1977) Alterations in the Function of the Nucleus Locus Coeruleus: a Possible Model for Studies of Anxiety. In *Animal Models in Psychiatry and Neurology*, I. Hanin and E. Usdin (Eds.). New York: Pergamon.

Redmond, D. E. (1979) The Effects of Destruction of the Locus Coeruleus on Nonhuman Primate Behaviors. *Psychopharmacology Bulletin* 15:26–27.

Redmond, D. E. (1983) Social Effects of Alterations in Brain Noradrenergic Function on Untreated Group Members. In *Hormones, Drugs, and Social Behavior in Primates*, H. Steklis, and A. Kling (Eds.). New York: Spectrum.

Redmond, D. E., Huang, Y. H., Snyder, D. R., Maas, J. W., and Baulu, J. (1977) Hyperdipsia After Locus Coeruleus Lesions in the Stumptailed Monkey. *Life Sciences* 20:1619–1628.

Sackett, G. P. (1966) Monkeys Reared in Isolation With Pictures As Visual Input: Evidence For an Innate Learning Mechanism. *Science* 154:1468–1472.

Siegelbaum, S. A., Camardo, J. S., and Kandel, E. R. (1982) Serotonin and Cyclic AMP Close Single K+Channels in Aplysia Sensory Neurones. *Nature* 299:413–417.

Suomi, S. J., Seaman, S. F., Lewis, J. K., Delizio, R. D. and McKinney, W. T. (1978) Effects of Imipramine Treatment of Separation-Induced Social Disorders in Rhesus Monkeys. *Archives of General Psychiatry* 35:321–325.

Suomi, S. J., Kraemer, G. W., Baysinger, C. M., and Delizio, R. D. (1981) Inherited and Experiential Factors Associated with Individual Differences in Anxious Behavior Displayed by Rhesus Monkeys. In *Anxiety: New Research and Changing Concepts* D. F. Klein and J. Rabkin (Eds.). New York: Raven Press.

Walk, R. C., Murphree, O. D., and Angel, C. (1976) A Multivariate Discriminate Analysis of Behavioral Measures in Genetically Nervous Dogs. *Pavlovian Journal of Biological Sciences* 11:175–179.

Walters, E. T., Carew, T. J., and Kandel, E. R. (1979) Classical Conditioning in Aplysia Californica. *Proceedings of the National Academy of Sciences* 76:6675–6679.

Walters, E., Carew, T. and Kandel, E. (1981) Associated Learning in Aplysia: Evidence for Conditioned Fear in an Invertebrate. *Science* 211:504–506.

5

Animal Models for Schizophrenia

Introduction

In many ways this was the most difficult chapter to write. Clearly, the group of psychiatric illnesses lumped under the overall term *schizophrenia* represents a major public health problem. Though it remains a puzzling illness, there have been major advances in our understanding of schizophrenia and in diagnostic conceptualizations.

However, from the standpoint of animal modeling, schizophrenia research has not kept pace with that in other areas (e.g., depression, anxiety disorders, alcoholism, etc.). The amount and variety of research activity have been quite limited. Indeed, serious questions have been repeatedly raised as to whether this is an area worth pursuing. Those who would question it point out that since schizophrenia is a thought disorder involving dysfunction of higher symbolic processes, perhaps it is a disease unique to humans; therefore, attempts to develop animal models are bound to prove fruitless. This issue is discussed in this chapter, and a review of past and current approaches to developing animal models of schizophrenia is provided.

Regardless of one's position on the above issue, it has proven difficult to develop measures of animal behavior and/or thinking that have face validity in relation to human schizophrenia. Most of the defining characteristics of human schizophrenia involve patients' descriptions of what they are experiencing. For example, we have no way to know if an animal is hallucinating, or having delusions or loose associations. Furthermore, there are fewer behavioral parameters used in the diagnosis of schizophrenia than there are in depressions or even in anxiety disorder. This makes animal modeling research in this area exceptionally difficult.

However, the creative deployment of animal models of specific aspects of schizophrenia could potentially assist greatly in unraveling the pathogenesis of this puzzling group of illnesses. What has been tried? Most of the work has involved the drug induction of altered behavior patterns, mainly stereotypic behaviors and/or hyperactivity, and their reversal by neuroleptic agents. In terms of drug screening, the models have what in previous chapters has been called high empirical validity. Most proposed animal models of schizophrenia have this as their major, if not only, validating criterion. One of the additional areas of animal modeling research in schizophrenia relates to arousal models, and these are also discussed in this chapter.

The reader should realize that this is not a highly developed area of research activity despite the creative efforts of a few individuals. Nevertheless, it is an area in which some new approaches are needed, and, in this chapter, suggestions are made in this regard.

Schizophrenia remains a puzzling, indeed enigmatic, form of psychopathology. Significant progress has been made in a number of research and clinical areas, yet our basic understanding of this devastating illness is still quite limited. There are, undoubtedly, major genetic determinants, but the mechanisms of these genetic influences and the nature of their interaction with developmental events, family and social events, and neurobiological substrates is largely unknown. Genetic vulnerability is important but only accounts for a certain proportion of the variance in the occurrence of most forms of schizophrenia. The pathogenesis of schizophrenia is largely unknown. It is possible to control many of the symptoms of schizophrenia with neuroleptic medications, but these have major and undesirable side effects, and there is clearly a need for improved experimental systems for developing medications that do not carry such great risks. The role of social and interpersonal therapies in a battery of approaches to treating schizophrenia is controversial, and there are limited data regarding how these approaches might be influenced by, or in turn influence, underlying neurobiological functioning.

The above are merely a few of the reasons for developing animal models of schizophrenia. Animal models are needed to investigate, in a controlled manner, the etiology, pathogenesis, and other specific aspects of these illnesses. Experimental systems in animals are also needed to develop improved psychopharmacological agents and to enable documentation of which behaviors are being affected in which way by specific drugs. Just as in the cases of depression, anxiety, and alcoholism, we should not try to develop global models of the schizophrenic syndromes in animals—this is impossible. However, by focusing the development of an experimental system on a specific aspect of the schizophrenia syndromes, it may be possible to develop some useful animal models. Certainly some of the work that must be done cannot be done in humans. Therefore, if useful experimental systems can be developed in animals, progress in this research area could be facilitated.

This chapter first briefly reviews those clinical aspects of schizophrenia which are most relevant to animal model development. Of course, this part of the chapter cannot be comprehensive since many volumes have been, and continue to be, written on this topic. It is therefore selective but, it is hoped, sets the clinical framework for consideration of specific approaches to development of animal models. This section of the chapter also contains a review of some historical as well as current approaches being used to develop animal models of schizophrenia. Finally, there is a discussion of some new approaches which might be considered as we move to a new era of animal modeling. These approaches are related to ongoing clinical research on the one hand, and to a growing ethological literature on the other. It is a challenge to combine these two in ways that have rarely been done in the past. Animals are not just miniature humans from which we can obtain certain measures in controlled living conditions in ways impossible to do in humans. It is true that we can often obtain certain measures, but if sufficient attention is not paid to the social context in which the measures are being obtained, the conclusions that can logically be drawn will be limited. Technological sophistication in neurobiology must be accompanied by an equal degree of sophistication in social behavior assessment. This is a recurrent theme in this chapter and others. As part of the excitement of this era of "high-technology neuroscience," behavioral studies and assessment techniques are sometimes being shortchanged. This is unfortunate. If the behavioral aspects of the models are not as sophisticated as the neurobiological aspects, the usefulness of animal models in enhancing our understanding of this utterly devastating clinical syndrome, as well as any other syndrome, will be sharply limited.

The Clinical Syndrome

There have been many books written on the clinical aspects of schizophrenia. Much of this section derives from a book by Strauss and Carpenter that presents a useful interactive model of schizophrenia

(Strauss and Carpenter, 1981). Of particular relevance for the discussion of animal models which follows are the principles which they present for understanding schizophrenia:

1. There is a group of behaviors and/or mental processes that can be specified and which distinguish schizophrenia from other psychiatric syndromes. This does not mean that they are unique to schizophrenia but that taken together they have a special association with schizophrenia. Some may overlap with other syndromes so that a single behavior in isolation does not a schizophrenic make. In other words, a given behavior or symptom alone may not be diagnostic, but when it occurs in the company of a cluster of other symptoms, it may be. Many examples of this principle come up in the review of animal models.

2. Schizophrenia is not a homogenous syndrome and probably consists of many subvarieties that may have different etiologies, pathogeneses, presentations, and treatments. Current diagnostic systems reflect this conceptualization and, in particular, distinguish the schizophrenias from closely related syndromes that either never develop into psychoses or are very brief and not followed by changes in function indicative of the more malignant forms of schizophrenia. The definition of psychosis and the duration issue must be included in the evaluation of schizophrenia models.

3. To have a comprehensive basis for understanding schizophrenia, genetic, biochemical, neurophysiological, social, cultural, developmental, and probably other mechanisms must be considered.

Obviously, animal modeling research cannot solve all of these issues, but, given this conceptualization of schizophrenia, there is room and need for a plurality of models. One model cannot encompass all the important aspects of the illness. Historically, the biggest mistake has been talking about a model for schizophrenia and then arguing how that particular model relates to the various aspects of the human syndrome. The position taken here is that animal modeling research in schizophrenia is at the stage where only modest claims about a given experimental system should be made. It is important to develop experimental systems in parallel and in some depth. The investigator studying, for example, stereotypic behavior following amphetamine administration in animals needs to study this in some depth but not overly generalize from the results to implications about the role of dopamine in schizophrenia in general; that is, there is a need to develop individual systems in depth but at the same time keep an overall perspective.

4. In the past, prognosis has been a part of the definition of schizophrenia. It is increasingly recognized that the prognosis is variable and can be influenced by a number of variables. Most proposed animal models are acute and have not dealt with this issue. However, as part of the study of experimental paradigms in animals, the study of the variables which influence the course would be indicated and have only rarely been done.

Clinical Diagnosis

This section is being included so the reader will have the criteria in mind when the various models are reviewed.

DSM-III Criteria for a Schizophrenic Disorder (Diagnostic and Statistical Manual, 1980)*:

1. At least one of the following during a phase of the illness:
   a. bizarre delusions
   b. somatic, grandiose, religious, nihilistic, or other delusions without persecutory or jealous content
   c. delusions with persecutory or jealous content if accompanied by hallucinations of any type
   d. auditory hallucinations (details specified in *DSM-III*)
   e. incoherence, marked loosening of associations, markedly illogical thinking, or marked poverty of content of speech if associated with at least one of the following:
      (1) blunted, flat, or inappropriate affect
      (2) delusions or hallucinations
      (3) catatonic or other grossly disorganized behavior
2. Deterioration from a previous level of functioning in such areas as work, social relations, and self-care.
3. Duration: Continuous signs of the illness for at least 6 months at some time during the person's life, with some signs of the illness at present. The manual gives further specification of what the 6-month period must include.

---

*Since this book was written, *DSM-III-R* (APA, 1987) was published; these revised criteria are essentially the same, although employing modified and expanded language.

4. If there was a manic or depressive episode, it must be brief in relation to the duration of the psychotic symptoms.
5. Onset before age 45.
6. Not due to any organic mental disorder or mental retardation.

DSM-III uses a modified multiaxial approach, and other systems have also been suggested (Strauss and Carpenter, 1981). Consistent with a current trend in psychiatry, *DSM-III* relies heavily on signs and symptoms and on prior duration. This is a source of considerable controversy, and others have suggested a multiaxial system that includes, in addition to symptoms and course, such things as associated life events, social relations function, and work function. This chapter does not deal with these diagnostic differences but rather extracts what is most relevant for various approaches to animal modeling.

Perhaps the most obvious is that schizophrenia is, by definition, a thought disorder, and assessment of many of the hallmark signs and symptoms requires verbal ability. This, of course, cannot be done in animals. It is impossible to know if an animal is delusional or hallucinating or if it has loose associations. Though an exhaustive review of the various diagnostic systems for classifying schizophrenic patients is beyond the scope of this chapter, it should be noted at the outset that there are no animal analogues or homologues available for many of the characteristic signs and symptoms of schizophrenia: auditory hallucinations, flatness of affect, thought alienation, thoughts spoken aloud, delusions of control, neologisms, associative disorders, ambivalence, and incongruous affect. Speculations have been offered regarding possible analogues for autism and for waxy flexibility.

The present lack of behaviors in animals that can be said to correspond to hallmark signs of schizophrenia should not discourage investigators from working on ways to make schizophrenic signs and symptoms operational. This will likely involve, on the one hand, a ethological analysis of human schizophrenia before proceeding to animal parallels. On the other hand, some limited but important aspects of human schizophrenia may be studied in animals without making overly exaggerated claims of similarity to the global syndrome.

Criteria for Evaluating Animal Models of Schizophrenia

Is it possible for a psychosis such as schizophrenia to be produced in animals? How are the proposed models evaluated? This general topic has been discussed in a previous chapter, but Matthyse and Haber (1975), pp. 5–6 have formulated some additional specific criteria with regard to schizophrenia. They are mostly drug related and are as follows:

1. "The aberrant animal behavior should be restored to normal, at least in part, by drugs which are known to be effective in the treatment of schizophrenia." As a subset of this criterion, they felt that the relative potencies of the various neuroleptics should also characterize their normalizing effects in the animal model.
2. Drugs which are related in chemical structure to the effective antipsychotic drugs, such as the phenothiazines and butyrophenones, but which have no effect in treating human psychoses, also ought not to work in the animal model.
3. Tolerance "should not develop to the behavior-normalizing effects in the animal model since it does not develop to antipsychotic drug action in humans."
4. "The normalizing effects of neuroleptics in the animal model should not be blocked by the simultaneous administration of anticholinergic agents." The logic behind this as a criterion is that anticholinergic agents are often used clinically along with neuroleptics without interfering with their clinical effects.

Matthyse and Haber describe these criteria as amounting to a requirement of "isomorphism in a mathematical sense." Each formal characteristic of one system is required to have an exact counterpart in another, although the objects contained in the two systems may not be alike. In this case, the two systems are the clincial syndrome of schizophrenia and the animal behavior selected as a model. The formal characteristics that are required to be preserved in going from one system to the other are the responses to pharmacological agents.

Basically, these are criteria to evaluate the empirical validity of the model in terms of predicting drug responsiveness across species. As will be seen, most proposed animal models of schizophrenia use this as the major, if not only, validating criterion. This may be as good as the present state of knowledge about human schizophrenia allows. Human schizophrenia has not been well described from a behavioral standpoint, nor are there any validating physiological criteria. The etiology is unknown. Perhaps if some good animal preparations for studying specific signs, symptoms, and/or behaviors that occur in schizophrenia can be developed, it may be possible to get some clues about the etiology of the syndrome itself.

Claridge (1978) called attention to four difficulties in creating an animal model of schizophrenia. First, he suggested that schizophrenia might be an entirely human condition, and that if this was so, the search for an equivalent in lower animals would be very difficult, if not fruitless. This view is held by those who consider disorders of language, thinking, and social communication to be the hallmark features of the disease and not present in animals. As Claridge points out, there are two ways to conceptualize a response to this difficulty. The first is to develop some features of schizophrenic thinking disturbances which can be measured in animals. This involves developing operational versions of the schizophrenic's thought disturbances. While work in this direction needs to be pursued, Claridge felt that, for the moment, our belief that animal models for schizophrenia are viable must rest on the assumption that the essential symptoms of schizophrenia, which themselves may not be modeled in animals, are derivative phenomena indicative of an underlying disturbance in neurobiological mechanisms; that is, certain core features of schizophrenia reflect disturbance of brain function and that these disturbances might be accessible in laboratory models. In this context, comparative research might help unravel one aspect of the schizophrenic illnesses. To be more specific, in animals we may be able to produce the hypothesized neurobiological deficits and study the effects of such alterations on social and cognitive behaviors.

The second problem Claridge pointed out was the difficulty in translating the core schizophrenic symptoms into a form that can be studied across species. He feels that this has not yet been done, and that the behaviors that have been studied, such as stereotypy following amphetamine administration, are not core features of the clinical syndrome.

The third difficulty is the heterogeneity in the behavior of human psychotic patients; that is, there are the schizophrenias rather than a single syndrome, and we are likely to need several animal models rather than any single comprehensive one.

A fourth difficulty is the failure of human clinical research to identify a unique set of defining parameters for schizophrenia. There are no reliable laboratory markers, and clinical diagnostic systems are in dispute. How can animal researchers model something so poorly defined?

Drug-Induced Models

Amphetamine and Psychostimulant Models

The amphetamine model is perhaps the best known approach to the experimental study of schizophrenia (Ellinwood, 1971; Ellinwood, Sudilovsky, and Nelson, 1973; Gambill and Kornetsky, 1976; Garver, Schlemmer, Maas, and Davis, 1975; Haber, Barchas, and Barchas, 1977;

Kornetsky and Markowitz, 1975, 1978; Kraemer, Ebert, Lake, and McKinney, 1983, 1984; Machiyama, Utena, and Kikuchi, 1970; Machiyama, Hso, Utena, Katagiri, and Hirata, 1974; Matthyse and Haber, 1975; Segal and Janowsky, 1978; Snyder, 1973; Trulson and Jacobs, 1979; Utena, 1974; Utena, Machiyama, Hso, and Katagiri, 1975). This model is based on the clinical effects of amphetamine in humans, the behaviors produced in animals following amphetamine administration, the known neurochemical effects of amphetamine, and the pharmacological dissection of the amphetamine syndrome in animals.

There is little doubt that amphetamine and other psychostimulants can produce psychoses in humans. There are many case histories of amphetamine psychosis in human misdiagnosed as paranoid schizophrenia. These have usually, though not always, occurred in the context of abuse of amphetamines. Although amphetamine psychosis and paranoid schizophrenia have many features in common, some clinicians feel there are important differences and that they can be distinguished (Ellinwood, Sudilovsky, and Nelson, 1973). Paranoid ideation, along with well-formed delusions, is a hallmark of amphetamine psychosis. The delusions may begin with vague suspicions followed by increased ideas of reference. Other amphetamine effects include heightened awareness, an acute sense of novelty and curiosity, overwhelming terror, stereotyped compulsive behavior, and possibly visual, auditory, and tactile hallucinations. Typically there is retention of clear consciousness and correct orientation. Individuals can be agitated and show "brisk" emotional reactions rather than being flat or apathetic. There are some differences from schizophrenics. Many features of the formal thought disorder are missing, and the affective components are quite different (i.e., the brisk emotional reaction rather than one that is flat and withdrawn). There are differences in the frequency of the types of hallucinations, though there is clear overlap. The point is that amphetamine psychosis and naturally occurring schizophrenia have great similarity in human, though there seems also to be some important differences.

There are a number of other interesting features of stimulant-induced psychosis in relationship to schizophrenia. Though anyone is potentially susceptible to becoming psychotic if the dose of stimulant is high enough and/or administered for long enough, those with a history of schizophrenia are more susceptible to lower doses for shorter periods. There are animal parallels to this "vulnerability" phenomenon (Kraemer *et al.*, 1984). However, certain schizophrenics seem to improve, rather than get worse, after low-dose psychostimulant administration, suggesting, along with other evidence, that there are at least two classes of schizophrenics that react differently to arousal.

What are the behavioral effects of amphetamine in animals? There are acute and chronic, progressive, and residual effects. These have been studied in a variety of animals including cats, rats, and monkeys (Ellinwood, 1971; Kornetsky and Markowitz, 1978; Machiyama et al., 1970; Machiyama et al., 1974; Segal and Janowsky, 1978; Snyder, 1973; Trulson and Jacobs, 1979; Utena, 1974; Utena, et al., 1975). One of the most frequently described behaviors is a marked increase in stereotypy. These are repetitive behaviors such as hand–eye probing, picking, walking in circles, etc. In most cases they are not entirely new behaviors; they are part of the animal's repetoire but become much more exaggerated following amphetamine administration. The exact form of the stereotypy is related to the species and probably also to the history of the individual animal. The stereotypies can be either social or solitary, though there is some evidence that with chronic administration, the solitary stereotypies come to predominate.

Other behavioral changes produced in animals by amphetamine include increased activity, frequent changes of visual field ("checking," or "hypervigilance"), and progressive social isolation. A number of studies (Garver, Schlemmer, Mass, and Davis, 1975; Haber, Barchas, and Barchas, 1977) describe these basic findings with some variation. Animals given amphetamine acutely do not sit still for very long. They are chronically active and on the move. While they are moving, they engage in a series of stereotypic behaviors which include such things as threatening, lip smacking, hand–eye movements, picking, sniffing, scratching, rocking, etc. In addition, they are constantly changing their visual field and scanning. There is typically a gradual reduction of such indices of social activity as proximity and grooming, and more time is spent in progressive social isolation. With continued administration, some species may develop postural fixation and/or a variety of dyskinesias. The stereotypic patterns can become more bizarre and constricted, and the self-grooming behavior may actually become mutilative.

Recent work indicates that many of the above effects of amphetamine are greatly exaggerated if there has been a history of social deprivation early in development, even if there have been many intervening years of normal social behavior prior to amphetamine administration (Kraemer et al., 1984). This type of early environmental experience, or the lack thereof, sensitizes the animal to later amphetamine administration and thus provides a paradigm wherein developmental experiences and neurobiology can be studied in relation to each other. Also, after amphetamine administration there are residual effects, and it is easy to reinstitute the earlier amphetamine-induced behaviors with a low dose of stimulant or perhaps even by conditioning techniques in some species. Thus, converging lines of evidence indicate that an earlier social experience at certain developmental stages can sensitize an animal to amphetamine's behavioral effects and also that a prior experience with amphetamine sensitizes an animal to later amphetamine administration. In this context, the amphetamine work is significant not so much in terms of whether or not a given effect is a reasonable animal model of schizophrenia, but in terms of offering a paradigm to investigate the interrelationships between a drug's effect on neurotransmitters and behavior and to what extent these effects are influenced by prior and/or current social experience.

It is the stereotypic behavior following amphetamine administration that has led to a series of other pharmacological studies. In general, drugs that have high antipsychotic properties in humans block amphetamine-induced stereotypy. This finding has been related to the possible dopaminergic mechanisms in schizophrenia, on the basis that amphetamine-induced stereotypy is mediated by increased dopamine turnover.

Some workers have tried to separate the stereotypic behavior from the increased locomotor activity produced by amphetamine. For example, Sever (1970) hypothesized that the stereotypic behavior was related to the release of striatal dopamine that is significantly increased with repeated amphetamine administration. By contrast, the increased locomotor activity is thought to be mediated by norepinephrine. Tolerance develops in locomotor activity with repeated doses of amphetamine, whereas tolerance does not develop in stereotypic behaviors. This approach attempts to distinguish the different types of amphetamine-induced behavioral alterations in animals and to elucidate the differential neurological mechanisms that may be involved.

Two other aspects of amphetamine models are interesting. Segel and Janowsky (1978), in a series of pioneering studies, reported the effects of *d*-amphetamine on behaviors in rats and have particularly focused on locomotor activity and stereotypy. They reported a progressive augmentation of both behaviors with repeated administration. It was not that the duration increased, but that the onset of stereotypy appeared more rapidly and the mannerisms were more intensified. By contrast, with increasingly larger doses administered acutely, the duration of stereotypy increased. These data were interpreted to mean that with long-term amphetamine administration there is a tendency toward increased preservation of progressively more focused and restricted behaviors. A similar phenomenon has been reported in rhesus monkeys (Kraemer, Ebert, Lake, and McKinney, 1984).

There is evidence that the behavioral effects of a number of drugs, including amphetamine, differ, depending on the social circumstances in which they are given. For example, Gambill and Kornetsky (1976) found that subordinate rats receiving *d*-amphetamine actively withdrew from social interactions, retreated to strategically defensible locations, and remained hypervigilant. By contrast, when the dominant rat received the maximum dose, it was totally oblivious to the other rats. They felt that the responses to drug treatment in subordinate rats may provide a model for the social behavior of frightened paranoid schizophrenics.

The major use of the amphetamine syndrome in animals has been to permit a pharmacological dissection of the different behaviors produced, especially stereotypy. Most data reported are consistent with the view that *d*-amphetamine produces stereotypies and hyperactivity via effects on the dopamine system, whereas the hypervigilant state may be produced by effects on norepinephrine systems. A critical question is to what extent we can generalize from the suggestion that these neurotransmitters are important substrates for particular behaviors to their possible role as important substrates for a broader range of behaviors, some of which may be characteristic of schizophrenia. Certainly, stereoypic behaviors and hypervigilance *per se* have no special relationship to schizophrenia and, indeed, are not even listed among the defining characteristics of the syndrome. They are undoubtedly typical occurrences in amphetamine-induced psychosis in humans, and so from this standpoint the animal studies provide a reasonable experimental system for modeling human amphetamine psychosis. They may also have high empirical value in terms of predicting clinical drug effectiveness. Furthermore, by doing careful pharmacological dissection of these behaviors, we may be able to more fully understand the basis for their occurrence in a broad range of psychiatric disorders. Thus, the work has value that transcends any controversial relationship with schizophrenia in particular, and the results of such studies should not be needlessly extrapolated to human schizophrenia in general.

Phenylethylamine Models

Another drug induction model uses phenylethylamine (PEA). This is a neuroamine that is an endogenous component of the mammalian brain and most highly concentrated in the limbic system of the human brain. For a number of reasons the suggestion has been made that it can produce an animal model of schizophrenia (Borosin and Diamond, 1978; Borosin, Havdala, and Diamond, 1977). First, PEA can induce stereotypies which mimic the amphetamine-induced stereotypies. It has been studied mostly in rats and involves such behaviors as increased exploratory activity and discontinuous sniffing, continuous head bobbing, remaining in one location for long periods of time, and not being distracted by loud noises. The main measures of stereotypic behavior reported seem to center on head movements, distractibility, and length of time the animal stays in one place.

Chronic administration of PEA can result in behavioral sensitization (i.e., shortened latency and increased duration of action), just as amphetamine can. Substitution of PEA for amphetamine, or vice versa, exactly maintains the form and intensity of the previously elicited stereotypies as well as the previously elicited sensitization phenomenon. Therefore, it is reasoned that similar mechanisms are indicated (i.e., brain dopaminergic mechanisms).

However, there are some differences. The duration of action of PEA is shorter than that of *d*-amphetamine, probably due to rapid metabolism by monoamine oxidase type B. PEA also has a shorter latency than *d*-amphetamine, and PEA-induced stereotypic behavior is more sensitive to blockade by neuroleptic agents, with very few extrapyramidal side effects. For example, clozapine and thioridazine are effective in much lower doses than in the *d*-amphetamine paradigm. Indeed, there is some evidence that PEA-elicited stereotypies are more specifically mediated via the mesolimbic system, for example, *d*-amphetamine (but not PEA) produces stereotypy when directly applied onto the neostriatum. Clozapine selectively blocks PEA behavior, and it is thought to be a more specific blocker in the mesolimbic system with fewer effects on the extrapyramidal system.

For the above reasons, some workers think that stereotypic behavior induced by PEA may be a more specific animal model for schizophrenia than that induced by amphetamine. It is interesting that when PEA stereotypy was compared with amphetamine-induced stereotypy, it was found that PEA stereotypy rather than amphetamine stereotypy was dependent on norepinephrine.

Thus we see illustrated two proposed animal models for schizophrenia based on drug-induced stereotypic behaviors. Other stimulant drugs have also been used in a similar manner. In a general sense, the major arguments that can be brought to bear for the validity of these models relate to the fact that clinically effective neuroleptic drugs reverse the stereotypic behaviors. While this kind of reasoning has a certain appeal, we must be cautious. From a theoretical standpoint, drugs could be reversing the stereotypic behaviors produced in animals by stimulants for reasons and by mechanisms that have nothing to do with why they work in human schizophrenia. Again, this does not mean that the reversal of amphetamine- or PEA-induced stereotypies might not be an effective drug screen or have high empirical validity in this context. However, we must be extremely cautious in saying, on the basis of this alone, as some have done, that this is an animal model of schizophrenia. Other aspects of the model must be considered. What do stereotypic behaviors have to do with human schizophrenia? Certainly they can be seen, but they are not pathognomonic in any sense of the term, nor are they typically included in anyone's list of diagnostic criteria. Thus the behavioral similarity criteria leaves much to be desired. Since the etiology and pathogenesis of schizophrenia remain a mystery, there are no validating criteria from these areas that can be applied. So the end result is that despite a large body of active and impressive research, there is not one biological finding that we can point to and insist that it is present in an animal preparation before the model is viable. This then is the problem that animal modeling researchers in schizophrenia face. What other approaches are being tried?

Hallucinogen Models

The use of hallucinogens, mainly LSD, to model schizophrenia in both humans and animals is not as fashionable today as it was in the 1950s through the 1970s (Bradley, 1957; Claridge, 1978; Key, 1956, 1964). Part of this probably involves science; part may involve the politics of science. In any case, there is legitimate scientific controversy regarding the similarities and differences of LSD-induced psychotic states and human schizophrenia. This chapter cannot review the details of this controversy, but there are good arguments both ways. Probably the more important reason is political and involves the current enchantment with dopamine theories of schizophrenia and the fact that amphetamine models are more suited to the study of such systems. However, in our rush to dopamine, we may have neglected an important body of work relating to attentional-filtering problems of schizophrenics, and what some are coming to think may be basic rather than derivative problems of arousal. This research area is complicated, and this book cannot do justice to the rapidly emerging data in this area. The point to be made is that we should not restrict our work with drug-induced models of schizophrenia to that which fits in with preconceived neurobiological theories. There is also an emerging psychological literature, and the use of drugs other than amphetamine to study such theories as arousal and attentional deficits is important for the future. The search for different animal paradigms should not be narrowed prematurely.

Noradrenergic Reward System Deficit

Stein and Wise (1971) have proposed that schizophrenia results in part from a defect of the noradrenergic reward system, produced by the accumulation of endogenously formed 6-hydroxydopamine due to a genetically determined enzymatic error. The theory that 6-hydroxydopamine is the aberrant metabolite that causes schizophrenia is based on animal studies which have shown that when injected alone into certain brain sites, 6-hydroxydopamine decreases stimulation and other rewarded behaviors. The effect of this treatment is long lasting. Furthermore, the behavioral deficits as well as the depletion of the brain norepinephrine induced by 6-hydroxydopamine are prevented by prior treatment with chlorpromazine.

Attempts have been made to relate this model system to the fundamental symptoms of schizophrenia as described by Bleuler (1911). He described the disturbances of association and affect and the diminution of emotional responsivity in the schizophrenic. If there were impairments of the reward systems, this would be interesting in terms of the affective blunting and inappropriate affect shown by such patients. This proposed model has had considerable heuristic value. One of the interesting things about this model is that it does take us beyond dopamine and it potentially taps into a broader range of cognitive–psychological phenomena of schizophrenia than the study of stereotypic behavior does alone.

Conditioned-Avoidance-Response Model

Historically, this has been the most widely used screening test for antipsychotic drugs (Kornetsky and Markowitz, 1975). In this procedure an animal is presented with a conditioned stimulus (CS), such as a buzzer or bell, which is followed after a specified interval by an unpleasant unconditioned stimulus (UCS), for example, footshock. A response during the interval between the CS and the UCS lets the animal avoid the shock. However, if the animal fails to respond and receives the UCS, then the same response allows it to escape the UCS. In other words, it can either avoid the noxious UCS altogether by responding during the interval between the CS and the UCS or escape from the UCS once it has started. Drugs are then tested and characterized according to their effects on these two kinds of responding—avoidance responding or escape responding. Typically, antipsychotic drugs selectively inhibit avoidance responding but leave escape responding intact. Drugs such as barbiturates do not have this kind of profile. They suppress avoidance responding only at doses that produce side effects (e.g., ataxia and sedation). Antianxiety drugs do not have a selective effect either. This kind of procedure effectively predicts clinical antipsychotic drug activity and has high empirical validity. The relationship of this procedure and its results to the pathogenesis of schizophrenia is unclear.

Arousal Models

One of the most exciting areas of schizophrenia research is in the area of arousal or attention. It is phrased in various ways, but it appears that a definite subgroup of schizophrenic patients suffers from the inability to filter out irrelevant stimuli. They appear to be in a state of chronic arousal and are unable to selectively attend. This may be a trait-related risk factor. Could it be studied experimentally in animal models? If so, then we would have an experimental system that could help unravel the pathogenesis of certain aspects of schizophrenia. Again, no one claims to have a model for all aspects of schizophrenia, but this phenomenon does seem to have held up as a core defect. Experimental analogues in animals would permit the study of this phenomenon in relation to genetic, developmental, and neurobiological factors in ways impossible to do in humans.

Kornetsky and Markowitz (1975) have pioneered the development of paradigms in animals to test concepts that are also tested in humans. In humans, several kinds of experimental tasks are used to assess these deficits. Two of the major ones are continuous motor performance and a more complex digit symbol substitution test which is actually a subtest of the Wechsler Adult Intelligence Scale (WAIS). Some additional detail about these tests is given to help the reader unfamiliar with this area appreciate the kinds of deficits being discussed. In the Continuous Performance Test (CPT) there are visual stimuli presented as letters. They are presented for 0.1 seconds with a 1.0-second interval between stimuli. One letter is designated as the "critical stimulus," and it is presented in a random fashion approximately every sixth or seventh presentation. The subject's task is to press a lever within the 1.1-second interval after the appearance of the critical stimulus, but not after any of the letters which are not critical stimuli. Errors of commission as well as errors of omission are possible. An error of commission occurs when the subject pushes a lever after a noncritical stimulus, an error of omission occurs when he fails to push a key after a presentation of a critical stimulus.

This CPT requires about 4–8 minutes of sustained attention. Brief lapses of attention show up as errors of omission.

The digit symbol substitution test (DSST) requires a brief 90-second cognitive effort and is generally not influenced by brief lapses of attention. It is a subsection of the WAIS and correlates very highly with overall WAIS scores.

The two tests seem to be related to different substrates and respond differentially to different classes of drugs. Drugs that affect higher cortical centers (e.g., barbiturates) differentially impair performance on the DSST, whereas chlorpromazine causes greater impairment on the CPT. It is thought that CPT performance is related to midbrain and brain stem structures.

What is the relevance of the above studies to schizophrenia and what has been done to develop such paradigms in animals? A number of investigators have suggested that there might be a primary dysfunction in the arousal system and in the subcortical areas that subserve arousal in the schizophrenic patient. Some evidence indicates that there may be a malfunction in the midbrain or brain stem reticular formation leading to an altered arousal system and attention impairment, that is, inability to maintain a "set" as in the reaction times experiments of Shakow and others (Kornetsky and Markowitz, 1975).

Can animal experiments be devised to model the putative hyper-arousal-induced deficit in attention? What was done was to electrically stimulate the mesencephalic reticular formation, while the animal was performing on the animal version of the CPT. The hypothesis was that stimulation would impair the animal's performance, and that chlorpromazine would attenuate this performance deficit. An inverted U-shaped curve was found; that is, as stimulation increased, performance was actually increased up to a point, but thereafter, with increasing stimulation, performance declined. Thus, stimulation of the reticular formation resulted in impaired performance after a certain point of stimulation, but chlorpromazine reversed this effect. It does appear that the effects of stimulation are specific for tasks requiring sustained attention. For example, if animals are trained on a fixed ratio or fixed interval reinforcement schedule, then stimulation has no effect. It remains to be seen how specific these effects are to the reticular formation as opposed to other brain regions and what the effects of a variety of drugs would be.

Kornetsky and Markowitz's summary of their work provides an appropriate ending for this chapter. The quote is lengthy, but it is included not only for its lucid summary of their specific work, but also

because of the perspective it provides on animal modeling of schizophrenia in general:

> . . . it is unlikely that an animal model for schizophrenia is possible;
> however, it is possible that some aspects of the disease state can be modeled.
>   Of the various behavioral models discussed, some may be no more than
> bioassays. The CAR [Conditioned Avoidance Response] seems to fall into
> this category. The procedure allows for the prediction of antipsychotic ac-
> tivity of drugs in patients, but it tells us very little about the disease process
> itself.
>   For a procedure to qualify as a model it need not mimic the disease in its
> entirety, but it must have some analogous relationship to a significant aspect
> of the disease that it models. The difficulty is that, give our present state of
> knowledge, we are not sure what constitutes the relevant or critical aspects of
> either the disease or the model. Chronic amphetamine abuse produces in
> man a paranoia-like state and stereotyped behavior. This drug-induced state
> has been offered as a model of paranoid schizophrenia. In animals
> amphetamine induces behavioral stereotypies. This drug-induced state is
> primarily a model of the drug-induced state in man, a model of a model. It
> may also be a model for the human disease. It is possible that the animal
> stereotypies and the paranoid ideation seen as the result of chronic
> amphetamine administration in man are parallel phenomena not related in
> an obligatory fashion, and that only the model paranoia is relevant to the
> disease. The drug-induced state in the animal may model either a relevant
> aspect or an irrelevant correlate of the relevant phenomenon in the human
> model. Considerable scrutiny of these amphetamine models is necessary
> before their applicability to schizophrenia can be accepted or rejected.
>   The proposed model of Stein and Wise, despite its logical consistency, is
> based on the unproven premise that schizophrenia is a disease in which the
> "reward system" is dysfunctioning. However, the model has generated a
> continuing series of experiments that should teach us a great deal about the
> neurochemistry of the "reward system."
>   The animal model that we have presented is based on the hypothesis
> that there is a dysfunction of the arousal systems in some schizophrenics.
> This hypothesis is, in turn, based on extensive experimental evidence that
> the core deficit in schizophrenic patients is an attentional one. Although the
> evidence for an attentional deficit in the schizophrenic is clear, the evidence
> that it is a core deficit, although compelling, is not conclusive. We may
> simply be modeling some unessential correlate of the disease, and our model
> may have only a peripheral relationship to the underlying basis of the dis-
> ease. If this is the case, then the model must, at a minimum, have some
> relevance in helping to understand the neural system under study. (1975, pp.
> 46–47)

Summary of Key Points

- *From a clinical standpoint, there are multiple reasons for developing
  animal models of specific aspects of schizophrenia. Clinical research advances document a major general basis for these disorders and significant*

neurobiological substrates. *However, the evidence is indirect, and if suitable animal preparations could be developed that have some behavioral similarities to human schizophrenia, the genetic and neurobiological hypotheses resulting from human research could be investigated in ways that complement human research.*

- *Also, by using higher-order animals with a repetoire of social behavior and with abilities to perform on various tests of cognitive function, we could investigate how developmental and social factors might interact with genetic and neurobiological vulnerabilities to produce disordered behavior and altered cognitive processing.*

- *We should not try to develop global models of the schizophrenic syndromes in animals. This is conceptually wrong and is bound to fail. Rather, we should focus on the development of specific experimental systems to investigate selected aspects of the human syndromes.*

- *Given a conceptualization of schizophrenia as involving genetic, biochemical, neurophysiological, social, cultural, developmental, and other mechanisms, a plurality of approaches to animal modeling in this area should be encouraged.*

- *The largest amount of work directed toward the development of animal models of schizophrenia involves drug-induced models, especially amphetamine and other stimulants. A variety of behavioral changes resulting from the administration of these agents have been described in animals. These include such things as increased activity, stereotypic behaviors, hypervigilance, and progressive social isolation. In general, drugs that have high antipsychotic potency in humans block stimulant-induced stereotypy. Thus, there is a set of drug-induced models that have high empirical validity in terms of drug screening. These types of models are also being used to do neurobiological studies of the substrates of such behavioral alterations.*

- *Another type of approach has focused on a possible noradrenergic reward system deficit in human schizophrenia. Based on this conceptualization, 6-hydroxydopamine has been used as a neurotoxin to alter this system in animals. There have been studies of the effects of psychoactive drugs in this paradigm.*

- *The conditioned avoidance response model has, historically, been the most widely used screening test for antipsychotic drugs. Again, this is a test with high empirical validity. The linkage with the pathogenesis of schizophrenia is unclear.*

- *A final, but potentially exciting, set of models is based on the finding that a subgroup of schizophrenics suffer from the inability to filter out irrelevant stimuli. They appear to be in a state of chronic arousal and are unable to attend. Attempts have been made to develop experimental systems in animals that will permit the study of this phenomenon in relation to genetic, developmental, and neurobiological factors in ways impossible to do in humans.*

References

Bleuler, E. (1950) *Dementia Praecox or The Group of Schizophrenias*, translated by J. Zin Ken. New York: International Universities Press.

Borosin, R. L. and Diamond, B. L. (1978) A New Animal Model for Schizophrenia: Interactions With Adrenergic Mechanisms. *Biological Psychiatry* 13:217–225.

Borosin, R. L., Havdala, H. S., and Diamond, B. I. (1977) Chronic Phenylethylamine Stereotypy in Rats: A New Animal Model for Schizophrenia. *Life Sciences* 21:117–122.

Bradley, P. B. (1957) The Central Action of Certain Drugs in Relation to the Reticular Formation of the Brain. In *Reticular Formation of the Brain*, edited by H. Jasper, L. Proctor, R. Knighton, W. Nowshay, and R. Costello. London: Churchill, pp. 123–149.

Claridge, G. (1978) Animal Models of Schizophrenia: The Case for LSD-25. *Schizophrenia Bulletin* 4:186–209.

Diagnostic and Statistical Manual III (1980). Washington, D.C.: American Psychiatric Association.

Ellinwood, E. H. (1971) Effect of Chronic Methamphetamine Intoxication in Rhesus Monkeys. *Biological Psychiatry* 3:25–32.

Ellinwood, E. H., Sudilovsky, A., and Nelson, L. M. (1973) Evolving Behavior in the Clinical and Experimental Amphetamine Model Psychosis. *American Journal of Psychiatry* 130:1088–1093.

Gambill, J. D. and Kornetsky, C. (1976) Effects of Chronic d-Amphetamine on Social Behavior of the Rat: Implications for an Animal Model of Paranoid Schizophrenia. *Psychopharmacology* 50:215–223.

Garver, D. L., Schlemmer, F., Maas, J. W., Davis, J. (1975) A Schizophreniaform Behavioral Psychosis Medicated by Dopamine. *American Journal of Psychiatry* 132:33–38.

Haber, S., Barchas, P. R., Barchas, J. D. (1977) Effects of Amphetamine on Social Behaviors of Rhesus Macaques: An Animal Model of Paranoia. In *Animal Models in Psychiatry and Neurology* I. Hanin and E. Usdin (Eds.). New York: Peregamon Press.

Key, B. J. (1956) Effect of LSD-25 on Potentials Evoked in Specific Sensory Pathways. *British Medical Bulletin* 21:30–35.

Key, B. J. (1964) Alterations in the Generalization of Visual Stimuli Induced by Lysergic Acid Diethylamide in Cats. *Psychopharmacologia* 6: 327–337.

Kornetsky, C. and Markowitz, R. (1975) Animal Models and Schizophrenia. In *Model Systems in Biological Psychiatry*, D. Ingle and H. Shein (Eds.). Cambridge, Massachusetts: MIT Press.

Kornetsky, C., and Markowitz, R. (1978) Animal Models of Schizophrenia. In *Psychopharmacology: A Generation of Progress*, M. Lipton, A. Dimascio, and K. F. Killam (Eds.). New York: Raven Press.

Kraemer, G. W., Ebert, M. H., Lake, R. and McKinney, W. T. (1983) Amphetamine Challenge: Effects in Previously Isolated Rhesus Monkeys and Implications for Animal Models of Schizophrenia. In *Ethopharmacology: Primate Models of Neuropsychiatry* New York: Alan R. Liss.

Kraemer, G. W., Ebert, M. H., Lake, R. L. and McKinney, W. T. (1984) Hypersensitivity to *d*-Amphetamine Several Years after Early Social Deprivation in Rhesus Monkeys. *Psychopharmacology* **82**:266–271.

Machiyama, Y., Utena, H., and Kikuchi, M. (1970) Behavioral Disorders in Japanese Monkeys Produced by the Long-Term Administration of Methamphetamine. *Proceedings of the Japan Academy* **46**:738–743.

Machiyama, Y., Hso, S. C., Utena, H., Katagiri, M., and Hirata, A. (1974) Aberrant Social Behavior Induced in Monkeys by the Chronic Methamphetamine Administration as a Model for Schizophrenia. In *Biological Mechanisms of Schizophrenia and Schizophrenia-like Psychoses*, H. Mitsuda and T. Fukuda (Eds.). Tokyo: Igakushoin Ltd.

Matthyse, S., and Haber, S. (1975) Animal Models of Schizophrenia. In *Model Systems in Biological Psychiatry*, D. J. Ingle and H. M. Shein (Eds.). Cambridge, Massachusetts: MIT press.

Segal, D. S., and Janowsky, D. S. (1978) Psychostimulant-Induced Behavioral Effects: Possible Models of Schizophrenia. In *Psychopharmacology: A Generation of Progress*, M. A. Lipton, A. D. Dimascio, and K. F. Killam (Eds.). New York: Raven Press.

Sever, P. S. (1970) Receptor Sensitivity in Schizophrenia. *Lancet* **2**:312.

Snyder, S. (1973) Amphetamine Psychosis: A Model of Schizophrenia Mediated by Catecholamines. *American Journal of Psychiatry* **130**:61–67.

Stein, L. and Wise, C. D. (1971) Possible Etiology of Schizophrenia: Progressive Damage to the Noradrenergic Reward System by 6-Hydroxydopamine. *Science* **171**:1032–1036.

Strauss, J. S., and Carpenter, W. T. (1981) *Schizophrenia*. New York: Plenum.

Trulson, M. E., Jacobs, B. L. (1979) Long-Term Amphetamine Treatment Decreases Brain Serotonin Metabolism: Implications for Theories of Schizophrenia. *Science* **205**:1295–1297.

Utena, Hiroshi (1974) On Relapse-Liability, Schizophrenia; Amphetamine Psychosis and Animal Models. In *Biological Mechanisms of Schizophrenia and Schizophrenia-like Psychoses*, H. Mitsuda and T. Fukuda (Eds.). Tokyo: Igakushoin, Ltd.

Utena, H., Machiyama, Y., Hso, S. C., Katagiri, M., Hirata, A. (1975) A Monkey Model For Schizophrenia Produced by Methamphetamine. *Contemporary Primatology*, 5th International Congress of Primatology. Basel: Nagoya 1974 Karger.

6

Animal Models for Alcoholism

Introduction

The final chapter in this section focuses on attempts to develop animal models of human alcohol abuse. A number of other topics could have been chosen for this, the fourth case example. Why alcoholism?

First, clinicians will easily recognize the magnitude of the clinical problem and the enormous difficulties in treatment of the disorders included under this diagnostic heading. Conceptual models, based on empirical data, regarding the etiology and/or pathogenesis of alcohol abuse syndromes are sorely lacking. Most would agree that multiple variables (e.g., genetic, developmental, social, neurobiological, personality structure, etc.) are involved, but the specifics of how they might interact to produce the final syndrome is largely unknown. Animal models are potentially useful in isolating single sets of variables, studying their impact, and then combining them to study how they interact. Such studies are virtually impossible to do in humans.

Second, there is an enormous literature and body of work centering on efforts to develop animal models of alcoholism. The work has been done in several species and uses widely varying experimental paradigms. This chapter provides a critical overview of this work in the context of the principles of animal modeling research discussed in previous chapters. Despite the large literature, there remains considerable skepticism among clinicians, as well as researchers in the area, about whether alcoholism can usefully be studied in animal subjects. A major proposition of this chapter is that such negativism arises out of ignorance of what animal models are, and are not, and a failure to be specific about what a given experimental paradigm can contribute to the overall research problem. This issue is perhaps best illustrated in controversies about the forced administration vs the voluntary consumption issue which is discussed in more detail later in this chapter.

The need to develop some basic principles for comparative psychiatry are thus illustrated extremely well in the case of alcoholism. It will become apparent that the problem, by and large, is not with the research itself. There are some exciting paradigms available for studying specific aspects of alcoholism. The problem is mostly with the interpretation of such studies at the conceptual level.

Clinicians, as well as researchers in this area, have been preoccupied with attempts to develop *an* animal model of alcoholism. Unrealistic and excessively broad criteria have been applied to almost all approaches, and the proposed models invariably fall short. There is no model that will meet all the criteria that have been proposed. Indeed, it may be rare that humans with an alcohol abuse problem meet all the criteria themselves. They may not even be a complete model of the syndrome that is being studied in animals—the ultimate of ironies!

As one reads through this chapter, particular attention should be paid to what are the specific contributions of each approach being tried in animals rather than focusing on how the paradigm being used in animals does not measure up to some set of unrealistic and inappropriate criteria. In the case of each paradigm, the clinician will recognize some similarities with human alcohol abuse problems as well as some differences. It is not surprising that this is so, with a syndrome as complicated as alcoholism with its many variables, each exerting main effects plus interactions. However, that is the nature of the syndrome(s) being studied in the case of alcoholism, and the continued development and study of a broad range of animal models in relation to specific aspects of this complicated clinical problem is strongly indicated in a spectrum of research approaches.

Nowhere is the need for principles of comparative psychiatry better illustrated than in experimental studies, in animals, of alcoholism. Despite a very large literature on this topic, there is a negative set toward this research area today. A frequently articulated position is that attempts to create animal models for human alcoholism have failed, and there is a pessimistic outlook regarding any further efforts. The theme of this chapter is that such an attitude is not justified and that the area has great potential if a more reasonable conceptualization of approaches to studying specific aspects of alcoholism in animals is developed. By and large, the problem is not with the research itself but with unrealistic and inappropriate criteria that models in this area have been forced to meet.

The central problem is that workers in the alcoholism modeling field, and others, seem to have been guided by attempts to develop a comprehensive animal model of alcoholism. Approaches that do not produce all aspects of alcoholism in a given animal preparation have been viewed as failures. There has been a focus on viewing differences between animal studies and human alcoholism as weaknesses of the model rather than important differences which themselves need to be understood. One still reads about efforts to develop a single animal model of alcoholism. In no other area of human psychopathology is one kind of animal preparation expected to be suitable for studying all aspects of the human syndrome. Why the difference in the case of alcoholism? Writers in this area still search for the elusive, all-inclusive model and, consequently, a definite note of nihilism appears in the literature, and in other circles, regarding alcoholism models.

Several workers over the years have proposed sets of criteria for "an animal model of alcoholism," and the following summary is an extraction of those rather than being identical to any one set. However, there are some common themes, many of which are incorrect (Lester and Freed, 1973; Mello, 1973, 1976).

Some have conceptualized animal models as miniature representations of the human syndrome, and any differences between the two were viewed as unfortunate. One of the most frequent criteria given is that the animal must voluntarily take alcohol orally, and that this must be done without food deprivation. Furthermore, alcohol must be the preferred liquid even in the presence of competing and desired fluids.

As part of the generally accepted criteria, the animal must also consume alcohol over a prolonged period and must have high blood alcohol levels. It must work to obtain alcohol even in the face of aversive consequences and become intoxicated over a prolonged period.

Most writers include in the list of criteria that the animal must develop tolerance to alcohol and must show physical dependence as evidenced by an abstinence syndrome upon withdrawal. In addition, many add the requirement that after abstinence there must be a reacquisition of drinking to intoxication and reproducibility of the alcoholic process. Furthermore, it must be shown that the physical dependence induced is due to the chronic administration of alcohol and subsequent removal, rather than to some kind of nutritional deficiency.

Most would even include the requirement that there be evidence that alcohol is serving as a reinforcer, for example, that animals increase the rate of operant responding in order to obtain alcohol. According to Lester and Freed (1973), "until it can be shown that the rat drinks alcohol for the same kind of central reinforcement that man seeks, then so-called animal models are merely phylogenetic analogues which bear only a superficial resemblance to man's alcoholism."

The remainder of this chapter reviews the major approaches to studying human alcoholism in animals. Historically, each approach has been evaluated against an unrealistic set of comprehensive criteria. Virtually all articles in this area suffer from this improper conceptualization, and I think this is why there is so much disillusionment and cynicism about animal studies of alcoholism. *There is no such thing as a comprehensive animal model of alcoholism, nor will there ever be.* The human syndrome itself is too complex, multidetermined, and variously manifested. Rather, a more useful conceptualization is as follows. We need a number of different animal preparations for studying specific aspects of a complex and heterogenous syndrome. A given animal preparation might be useful for studying one specific aspect of human alcoholism but totally useless for studying another aspect. This does not invalidate the preparation; rather, it sets some realistic limits. As the given approaches are reviewed, these general points are illustrated. However, one example can be given at this point. In studying physical dependence issues, it may not be necessary for the animal preparation to voluntarily self-select alcohol. Forced administration might accomplish the same thing. Indeed, such preparations are available and have contributed important data regarding the time course and some of the biological parameters involved in developing dependence as well as the course of withdrawal. Of course, such an animal preparation would be useless for determining alcohol preference under experimental stress paradigms, but the latter might not reveal anything about the development of physical dependence. It is a bit mysterious why these seemingly obvious points have not pervaded alcoholism research in animals to the extent they have in other experimental studies of psychopathology in animals. Of course, from an idealistic standpoint, everyone wants an animal preparation in which there is as close a relationship as possible to the human syndrome in terms of genetics, etiology, course, phenomenology, mechanisms, and treatment responsiveness. However, the degree of complexity of most human psychopathological syndromes, including alcoholism, is such that we must settle for much more limited animal preparations and desist from insisting on comprehensive preparations. The possible development of any general principles about human alcoholism from studies in animals will only unfold gradually and in limited and specific ways from such focused studies.

Meisch (1977, 1982) and Cicero (1980) have written excellent reviews of the methods used to study alcoholism in animals, and the reader is referred to these and to the references contained therein for more detail than is possible to present in this chapter. I am indebted to these reviews for a part of the organization of the section of this chapter dealing with approaches, though I have tried to discuss this area from a different perspective. The perspective is that of someone interested in animal behavior, especially primate social behavior, and the philosophical and conceptual issues involved in using animal preparations to study human psychopathology.

Genetic Studies

It is clear from a number of studies that strains of mice can differ in their spontaneous consumption of alcohol. Selective breeding programs have been successfully conducted. Some strains drink very little, while others will drink almost as much alcohol as they can metabolize. This approach is exemplified in studies in Finland in the research laboratories of Alko (Eriksson, 1968, 1980), where they have produced two strains, the AA strain which consumes considerable alcohol, and the ANA strain which drinks very little. The strategy is to study biochemical, physiological, and behavioral differences between mice strains selectively bred for differences in alcohol intake. As Meisch (1982) says, a number of differences have been identified, but whether these differences have anything to do with differences in alcohol intake is an unsettled question.

Riley and colleagues (1976, 1977) reasoned that, based on the work going on in Finland since 1963, there was clearly a genetic contribution to the self-selection of alcohol but that such voluntary self-selection did not necessarily bear any relationship to the consequences of alcohol intake. That is, the increased consumption of alcohol shown by some rat strains was not a result of the effects of alcohol. These researchers selectively bred rats and used several dependent measures in addition to oral selection of alcohol as a phenotype. They tried to develop rat strains which exhibited extremes of reactivity to subhypnotic doses of alcohol in hopes of developing one strain in which a given dose of alcohol would have minimal effect and another in which the same dose would produce evidence of intoxication. They bred through several generations and found they could indeed separate two strains of rats differing in their reactivity to subhypnotic doses of alcohol. The dose issue is important to keep clearly in mind. The interesting point is that subhypnotic doses could have different effects in different species. It would be no accomplishment to produce intoxicating effects in all species with high enough doses, but the ability to find differential effects at a given subclinical dose is important. This is probably due to an interaction between genetic predisposition and does. The dependent measures used were impairment of motor coordination and equilibrium, and the two lines were designated "most affected" (MA) and "least affected" (LA). By the ninth generation, the LA animals showed 4 times as much activity as the MA animals after alcohol. The two lines differed only on the two dependent measures. This behavioral difference in response to a given dose of alcohol was not reflected in blood alcohol concentration, alcohol intake, or alcohol self-selection. The two lines also responded similarly on tests of emotionality.

Li, Lumening, McBride, and Waller (1979) selectively bred rats that would voluntarily drink enough alcohol to produce a central nervous system effect. Through 13 generations they were able to accomplish this and to produce high-drinking animals whose drinking was voluntary and not dependent on caloric restriction. They found that the animals would work to obtain ethanol, even when food and water were freely available, and were relatively insensitive to the hypnotic or sedative effects of ethanol, that is, they were tolerant. The amount of ethanol voluntarily consumed approached the animals' maximum capacity for ethanol elimination. Furthermore, this amount of ethanol consumption was capable of altering brain neurotransmitter content. These same animals would also work, by bar pressing, for the intravenous administration of ethanol. With prolonged free-choice consumption, ethanol intake increased to as much as 12 g/kg/day without producing overt behavioral deficits, further supporting the fact that these animals were tolerant. These rats were presented as a "model" for investigating the interaction of genetic, metabolic, and environmental factors in the production of alcoholism. Rephrased in the idiom of comparative psychiatry, researchers have been able to breed genetically susceptible rats which can then become an experimental animal preparation for studying how different environmental and pharmacological events might differentially influence the drinking behavior of this line in contrast to a line of rats which is not genetically susceptible.

Given the (by now well established) fact that selective breeding can produce strains of mice and rats that will consume higher quantities of alcohol than others and show differential effects to a given dose, what is the mechanism of these differences? Rodgers (1972) and Drewek and Broadhurst (1981) have used the term "genetic architecture" and have asked about the nature of the genetic variation controlling the phenotype. They did a triple testcross analysis of alcohol preference to learn about the gentic architecture of alcohol preference among male rats. Using mathematical calculations, they found directional dominance for low alcohol consumption but not for high alcohol consumption. Since dominance was for low, but not for high, alcohol preference, they reasoned that the heterozygosity present among noninbred subjects would result in low phenotypic levels of alcohol drinking, thereby precluding drinking to intoxication. To avoid this effect of dominance, certain inbred strains which display appropriate additive genetic properties may be used as part of selective breeding to produce high-drinking strains.

Rodgers (1972) and Rodgers and McClearn (1962) have also studied factors underlying differences in alcohol preference of inbred strains of mice. In one study they reported that the strain, or genotypic variable, accounted for over 97% of the total variance in alcohol consumption, with such things as error of measurement, sex differences, age differences (litter effects), and combined other effects accounting for less than 3% of total variance. They made the important point that some mouse strains normally consume alcohol to almost metabolic capacity under nonstressful conditions. Given this high baseline, it becomes very difficult to demonstrate a further increase as a result of experimental stress procedures ("the high-baseline effect"). Thus, if we are interested in evaluating the role of specific stressors on drinking behavior in animals, we would need to use a line (or a species) whose alcohol consumption was well below peak metabolic capacity. As we read the literature, it becomes apparent that this has not always been done, and, as a result, there may have been some false negative results concerning the possible effect of certain stressors on drinking behavior.

By way of summary, it can be said that by selective breeding of rats and mice, it is possible to produce animal preparations for high and low alcohol consumption. It is not known to what extent genetic variation may influence drinking behavior in higher-order animals, though it seems clear in the case of humans that genetic factors are important variables in alcoholism. The mechanisms underlying these genetic influences are completely unclear. Furthermore, very little is known about how genetic vulnerability interacts with developmental influences to produce increased alcohol consumption. These are all questions that could be investigated in specific animal preparations if the preoccupation with demanding only comprehensive preparations could be circumvented. Such preparations might tell us very little about dependence or withdrawal yet contribute important data without having to meet the constraints of unrealistic broad criteria. For example, is it possible that genetically vulnerable animals are influenced in their alcohol preference by exposure at certain developmental stages, but that animals which are not genetically vulnerable do not develop the alcohol preference even with exposure at the same developmental stages? These kinds of interactions are complex and virtually impossible to investigate in a controlled manner in humans, hence, the special value of animal preparations to study specific and important clinical questions in special ways. It may be, as Meisch says (1982, 1977), that there are no reports of high-intake strains drinking enough ethanol to develop physiological dependence or to show disruption in their ongoing behavior. However, under conditions of exposure to certain kinds of stressors, such strains might react differently in important ways, even though they might not be different under baseline conditions. This is an important interaction that can be investigated in animals.

Techniques Used to Induce Animals to Self-Administer Alcohol

Introduction

The technique most frequently used to induce animals to self-administer alcohol involves letting an animal have a choice between two drinking bottles presented concurrently, one containing ethanol and the other containing another solution, most commonly water. This technique has the advantage of simplicity and economy, but there are a number of technical problems regarding the use of the bottles themselves as well as with data analysis. The review of the technical details, beyond the scope of this chapter, is included in several of the chapter references (e.g., Amit, Amir, and Corcoran, 1973; Meisch, 1977; Myers, 1966; Myers and Holman, 1966; Wayner and Fisher, 1973).

Other paradigms involve the use of liquid dippers which can present precise volumes of liquid for prescribed durations. Responding on an operant task, for example, can be intermittently reinforced by access to the dipper cup. This permits recording of temporal pattern of intake but also data about other dependent variables such as the number of responses and reinforcements (Meisch and Thompson, 1971; Mello and Mendelson, 1964; Myers and Carey, 1961).

Additional techniques involve self-administration intragastrically through an indwelling nasogastric catheter (Amit and Stern, 1969; Yanagita and Takahashi, 1973) or intravenously (Deneau, Yanagita, and Seevers, 1969; Winger and Woods, 1973; Woods, Ikomi, and Winger, 1971). These obviously eliminate the taste factor and permit delivery of exact amounts of alcohol. Many writers cite as drawbacks the fact that humans self-administer alcohol orally rather than intravenously or intragastrically. This criticism represents a fundamental misunderstanding in that we do not have to duplicate all aspects of the human clinical situation in all animal paradigms for the work to be useful. The appropriate technique of administration depends on what we are studying. Many studies relevant to human alcoholism might conceivably be best done in animals who are self-administering intravenously or intragastrically, whereas other studies are best done in animals who are self-selecting oral administration of alcohol.

Electrical Stimulation and Intracerebral Injections

In one of the earliest series of studies, ethanol was injected directly into the lateral ventricle of rats for varying periods of time and at different concentrations. The rats were then tested in an alcohol preference test (Myers, 1964). There was a dose–response relationship between the intraventricular amount of ethanol and the amount taken orally. These intracerebral injections of ethanol were done in animals which normally did not select even low ethanol concentrations, and the amount of ethanol that was injected was of such minute proportions that there were no systemic or ingestive properties. Following chronic injections of several doses of ethanol for 10 days, increases in preference for ethanol occurred and were directly related to the dose of intracranial ethanol given. One proposed conclusion, based on these studies, is that a cellular biochemical change takes place in the brain stem with prolonged ingestion of ethanol, and this change may be the factor which governs voluntary ethanol consumption, rather than any effects of the alcohol *per se*, since there were no apparent effects in the animals in this paradigm.

Electrical stimulation of the lateral hypothalamus is another technique that has been studied with regard to whether or not it would lead to increased alcohol consumption (Wayner and Greenberg, 1972; Wayner, Greenberg, Carey, and Nolley, 1971). It has been found that 30 stimulation events over a period of 45 minutes induced consumption of alcohol concentrations as high as 20% at dose levels comparable to those observed during schedule-induced polydipsia (to be described below). The animals were described as grossly intoxicated, but they did not develop physical dependence after 25 days of exposure to lateral hypothalamic stimulation. Mello (1973) contrasts this to the dependence produced after multiple daily polydipsia sessions in which there are sustained high blood alcohol levels. Also, lateral hypothalamic stimulation did not induce preference for alcohol in the home cage situation. This approach, involving electrical stimulation of the hypothalamus, has been severely criticized because the animals do not develop a continuing preference for alcohol and do not become physiologically dependent. Such criticisms are unfounded. Why should we have to work on all of these parameters in one model? Different preparations will likely be needed for each. It is of great interest to determine which brain areas, when stimulated, result in increased alcohol intake even if only on an acute basis. Chronic alcohol intake with physiological dependence is not the only form of alcoholism. The magnitude of the increased ethanol drinking seen in this paradigm as well as the factors responsible for the increase are matters of some controversy. In one report the implantation of stimulating electrodes into the lateral hypothalamus of rats depressed ethanol intake as compared to unimplanted control rats. When they were stimulated, the ethanol intake increased, but only up to the level of unoperated control rats. Wayner and Greenberg reported that the electrical stimulation of the hypothalamus, while it can result in an increase in ethanol consumption (1.0 mg/kg/day), is not as powerful as periodic withdrawal of ethanol (presenting ethanol every other day), which results in an increased consumption of about 4.0 g/kg/day (Wayner and Greenberg, 1972). However, in this type of preparation it is eminently feasible to eliminate the problem of reduced food intake. This is done by utilizing preparations in which one pair of lateral hypothalamic electrodes produces drinking and another pair on the opposite side of the hypothalamus produces eating behaviors. Thus, the possible interrelationships of the effects of brain stimulation and the schedule of ethanol presentation are complex. Brain stimulation *per se* may have an effect, but so does the factor of intermittent alcohol availability.

    In a related vein is the work and theoretical conceptualization of Newman and colleagues (1980, 1983) on what they call "disinhibitory psychopathology." This involves lesions of the SHF system (medial septum, hippocampus, and prefrontal cortex) in animals. They find that rats with these lesions are less likely to delay gratification when given a choice between waiting 10 seconds for an assured reinforcement and an immediately available, though infrequently delivered, reinforcement. They speculate that there are disinhibitory syndromes in humans, including psychopathy, hyperkinesis, and alcoholism, and that septal-lesioned rats are a model for these syndromes, in that rats with these lesions are less able to defer rewards. In other words, rats with septal lesions will choose the immediately available, but less attractive, alternative, even when a capacity for behavioral inhibition was not required to select the more attractive but delayed alternative. There is an interesting theoretical paper on this subject (Gorenstein and Newman, 1980), but I am not aware of any specific data regarding alcohol consumption in such preparations.

Schedule-Induced Polydipsia

In 1961 Falk reported a technique in which food-deprived rats have intermittent access to dry food. (Falk, 1961, 1969; Falk and Tang, 1980; Meisch, 1977, 1982; Riley, Lotter, and Kolkosky, 1979; Wallace and Singer, 1976). Under these circumstances they will consume as much as one-half of their body weight in water within a few hours. Polydipsia is established with water, and then increasing concentrations of ethanol are substituted for the water. For example, the alcohol concentration can be increased by 1% increments every 6–8 days until 5–6% solutions are reached. This results in an ethanol intake of between 11 and 15 g/kg/day and blood levels above 100 mg/100 ml and usually between 150–300 mg/100 ml. The increased water intake seen under schedule-induced polydipsia does not persist when the food reinforcement is eliminated. However, if rats or rhesus monkeys have experienced drinking ethanol under these conditions, they will persist even after the concurrent food reinforcement is eliminated, thus suggesting that this paradigm results in ethanol serving as a positive reinforcer.

After 3-months exposure in this kind of paradigm and then abrupt withdrawal, withdrawal symptoms develop. Lester was the first to show that the polydipsia procedure was effective in producing intoxication in rats, and several other investigators have reported high levels of alcohol intoxication using a schedule-induced polydipsia paradigm, but none showed dependence until the Falk study described above.

The advantage of the schedule-induced polydipsia paradigm is that it is possible to maintain high levels of alcohol intake in the presence of adequate food intake, since animals can be maintained between 80 and 85% ad lib weight. The paradigm has been criticized on the basis that human alcoholics do not necessarily consume alcohol under these kinds of conditions. In other words, the incuding circumstances might be different across species. This might be true but does not invalidate the paradigm as a method to study the effects and consequences of schedule-induced drinking, including intoxication and withdrawal as well as the maintenance of drinking behavior.

Schedule-induced polydipsia is the only instance of physical dependence occurring in animals when alcohol is taken orally and electively. In general, taste-aversion learning limits the oral consumption of alcohol by animals, and thus blocks the development of physical dependence. However, by the use of some specialized procedures (e.g., schedule-induced polydipsia), it is possible to circumvent the taste-aversion limitation (Baker and Cannon, 1982). It is possible, using a liquid diet procedure, in which mice are food depleted and get 35% of their calories from ethanol, to get evidence of gross intoxication and physical dependence. However, apart from such dietary manipulations, it is difficult to establish alcohol as a reinforcer when it is taken orally. Two reasons for this have been given. The first is the aversive taste, and special training procedures are required to deal with this. The second is the delay between the drinking of alcohol and the onset of its interoceptive effects.

Intravenous Self-Administration

In contrast to the difficulty in establishing the reinforcing properties of oral alcohol, intravenous alcohol is clearly a reinforcer in animals. For example, monkeys can become addicted to alcohol using a paradigm in which they press a lever to activate an automatic intravenous injection apparatus. Deneau *et al.*, (1969) first demonstrated this phenomenon, and it has since been confirmed and extended by others (Winger and Woods, 1973; Woods *et al.*, 1971; Yanagita and Takahashi, 1973). The initiation of intravenous self-administration of alcohol does not occur as consistently as with cocaine and opiate narcotics. The reasons for this are not known, but if a high response rate is first established with cocaine or pentobarbital and then ethanol is substituted, it is easier to get monkeys to self-administer alcohol.

Monkeys will self-administer intravenous alcohol to the point of intoxication, and during the course of self-administration they will lose weight, decrease food intake, and show general ill health associated with malnutrition. Once they begin self-administration, the daily intake remains constant and tolerance does not develop. There may be episodes of self-imposed abstinence if they are given 24 hours per day access, but not over 3-hour test periods. These 3-hour test periods also do not produce physical dependence.

Again, the obvious fact that humans self-administer alcohol orally rather than intravenously has frequently been cited as a shortcoming of this paradigm. However, there are a number of very important questions that can be investigated in this paradigm and others that cannot. The fact that the drug gets in through the veins rather than through the gastrointestinal tract should not deter investigators as long as the differences are recognized and undue inferences not drawn. Mello cites a number of important questions regarding the maintenance of drug administration that could be investigated in this paradigm, even though it is not identical to the human syndrome. For example, there is some cyclicity to drug administration in animals and in humans. Why? Relatively little attention has been paid to the schedules of reinforcement which produce alcohol self-administration, and this kind of paradigm could be very helpful here. Also, the contribution of the condition of physical dependence to the reinforcing properties of alcohol is unclear.

Intragastric Self-Administration

This paradigm has considerable overlap with the above section on intravenous administration except that the alcohol is self-administered intragastrically through an indwelling nasogastric catheter. This eliminates palatability factors and permits delivery of precise amounts of alcohol (Amit and Stern, 1969).

Restriction of All Liquid to Ethanol Solutions

In this paradigm the animal has access to solid food, but the only liquid available is ethanol. No signs of intoxication or physiological dependence has been observed in rats or infant monkeys under these conditions.

What happens to ethanol intake under choice conditions after a period of restriction to ethanol? Both increases and decreases have been reported with the differences in results perhaps being due to the nature of the ethanol solution to which the animals were originally exposed. If the original solution was 7%, they subsequently drank more ethanol later under free-choice conditions. If the original solution was 15–20% they drank less ethanol under later free-choice conditions.

Forced Administration followed by Free Choice

In this paradigm, the animals are force-fed alcohol for a period of time and then later tested in a free-choice situation. For example, Deutsch and Walton (1977) presented an alcoholism model in which Charles river rats were force intubated with alcohol for 3 weeks and then subsequently tested in a free-choice situation. They consumed significantly more ethanol in the free-choice situation than rats which had been intubated with water. In this study, taste and smell of alcohol were eliminated as factors controlling intake. A number of the alcohol-intubated animals were subsequently reintubated and tested. They showed further increases in voluntary alcohol intake and a 70% preference for the alcohol-paired flavor, suggesting that relief of withdrawal symptoms was a major factor responsible for the increased alcohol ingestion following forced intubation.

Another technique is to force rats to drink a 1.7% saline solution to which various amounts of ethyl alcohol are added. The alcohol can then be withdrawn at various times. Dramatic and quite large amounts of drinking occur in the animals which had the alcohol added and then withdrawn, suggesting that the copious drinking of the saline solution can be attributed to the prolonged ingestion and withdrawal of the ethyl alcohol. Control groups which had had nonalcoholic vehicles added to the saline solution and then withdrawn did not show the increase in drinking. The authors discussed this work in terms of its implication as a means of inducing alcoholism in the rats, that is, forced drinking of saline plus ethyl alcohol (Waynerm Barone, and Jolicoeur, 1978).

In an earlier report, attempts had been made to artificially induce ethanol dependence in rhesus monkeys and then to assess their subsequent preference for ethyl alcohol (Myers, Stoltman, and Martin, 1972). In this study, successive preference–aversion functions in an ethanol–water choice situation were obtained for four rhesus monkeys. Each preference sequence consisted of a 9-day period during which the concentration of the ethanol solution offered to the animal was increased systematically from 3% to 30%. During the second and third ethanol preference sequences, a total of 6 g/kg ethanol was administered daily. Signs of physical dependence on ethanol were exhibited during the second intubation sequence, and severe symptoms of withdrawal occurred upon the termination of intragastric ethanol. Despite this, none of the monkeys increased volitional intake of ethanol during the final sequence.

Experimental Stressors and Alcohol Intake in Animals

A number of workers have recently called for increased attention to this area as one possible approach to studying an important aspect of human alcoholism, namely, the interaction between certain types of stressors and alcohol intake (Myers and Veale, 1972; Pohorecky, 1981).

In an early study, Masserman and Yum (1946) reported that cats often developed a definite preference for a solution of alcohol in milk if they were given alcohol during a conflict-conditioning procedure. Clark and Polish (1960) used two rhesus monkeys and determined measures of intake of water or of a solution of 20% alcohol in water before, during, and after avoidance conditioning. The specific conditioning involved the animals being trained to press a lever to avoid electric shock. Alcohol consumption increased during, and decreased after, avoidance sessions. Water intake remained the same or decreased during avoidance sessions and stayed at this level after the sessions.

Mello and Mendelson (1966, 1971) reported on the factors affecting alcohol consumption in primates. They studied four rhesus monkeys using avoidance conditioning, punishment, and free-choice experience. By punishment they meant the intermittent presentation of a noxious, unavoidable electrical shock. This had no effect on ethanol consumption in their paradigm. In the case of avoidance conditioning there was no increase in consumption for a monkey that refused ethanol in a free-choice situation. However, for a monkey that selected ethanol in the free-choice situation, there was a rapid increase in consumption associated with avoidance conditioning. This increase persisted for 75 days following termination of conditioning. There were no signs of withdrawal after abrupt removal, suggesting that there was no physiological dependency.

Rhesus monkeys have a strong aversion to alcohol. When confronted with a situation in which avoidance of a noxious shock is contingent upon a consumatory response, they are smart enough to learn a dual avoidance response (i.e., make the lick response required to avoid shock but yet have very little fluid dispensed).

In general, conditions that involve physical stress do not lead to a higher selection of alcohol. Conditions that involve uncertainty do lead to a higher selection of alcohol as compared to nonstress situations (Cicero, Myers, and Black, 1968; Orloff and Masserman, 1975, 1978).

A series of articles by Pohorecky and colleagues (1977, 1981) has reexamined this relationship between stress and alcohol. These articles are reviewed in a bit more detail because they contain important considerations about future work in this area.

The interaction between stress and alcoholism is complicated and not easily investigated even in animal subjects. Yet, if interesting paradigms can be developed to study this aspect of alcohol consumption in animals, there is much of clinical relevance to be learned. It is not necessary that the animals become physically addicted and have extremely high blood alcohol levels and withdrawal symptoms to appreciate the value of studying this aspect of the alcohol preference and abuse problem.

Typically, researchers have relied on such paradigms as conditioned avoidance, in which an animal must learn to make a response (e.g., choose alcohol) to avoid or turn off electric shock or some other noxious stimulus. This fits under the general heading of using stressors to get the animal to consume alcohol. Another approach involves the study of the effects of ethanol on subjects subjected to other stressors, and yet a third paradigm involves the effects of stressors in intoxicated subjects. All three approaches involve studying separate facets of the alcohol syndromes. In the literature, these distinctions have not often been made, until some recent articles by Pohorecky and colleagues called these key distinctions to everyone's attention. Again, failure to properly conceptualize this aspect of alcoholism research in animals has led to a sense of nihilism despite a number of very exciting approaches to studying this interface between stress and alcoholism.

Effects of Stressors in Intoxicated Subjects

It is widely thought that in intoxicated humans, stressors are supposed to have a sobering-up effect (the amethystic effect). However, there have been very few experimental studies on this subject. These have recently been summarized and generally indicate that stressors (e.g., metrazol, forced swimming, or prior inescapable shock) can partially reverse or prevent the depression produced by ethanol on various behavioral and physiological measures.

Ethanol Effects in Stressed Subjects

This approach is based on the early studies of Masserman and Yum (1946) and Conger (1956), who suggested that ethanol might improve the performance of stressed animals. In addition, some literature on humans suggests that ethanol might have beneficial effects in non-alcoholic subjects. In the Masserman and Yum work, cats were subjected to experimental procedures involving motivational conflicts between hunger and fear. Their conclusions were as follows:

> Under such circumstances they developed "experimental neuroses" characterized by pervasive inhibitions of normal goal responses, hypersensitivity and aversions to stimuli associated with the conflictual field, loss of group dominance, and marked and persistent aberrations of somatic and motor function. The administration of small doses of alcohol again disintegrated these relatively complex "neurotic" patterns and permitted relatively

simple goal-oriented responses to supervene. A significant number of animals who repeatedly experienced such relief from neurotic tensions developed a definite preference for alcoholic drinks, i.e., showed evidences of addiction to alcohol. However, as their re-exploratory behavior while mildly intoxicated partially resolved conflicts, this addiction diminished until nearly normal food choices were restored. (1946, p. 52)

One of the earliest studies cited by Pohorecky regarding this interaction examined the interaction of ethanol with audiogenic seizures and found that alcohol would protect against these seizures (Greenberg and Lester, 1953). Mildly sedative doses of ethanol (0.03%) prevented the occurrence of seizures in 42% of the trials, and blood levels of ethanol of 0.08% prevented seizures in all trials. An interesting finding in this regard is that of Dember and Kristofferson (1955) of a relationship between preference for ethanol and seizure susceptibility. Rats with the highest intake of 5% ethanol had the greatest susceptibility to seizures. Pohorecky *et al.*, (1981) questioned whether this finding said anything about the relationship of voluntary ingestion of ethanol and the level of central nervous system excitability. One possibility is that the higher intake of ethanol should have lowered the level of central nervous system excitability, and the voluntary intake may be limited by a homeostatic mechanism which also regulates the susceptibility to seizures. Intake of 10% ethanol in mice prevented the cardiomegaly produced by a choice audiogenic stressor.

At the behavioral level, most experimental research has provided inconclusive or contradictory results for an interaction of stressors with ethanol. In general, ethanol restores a normal pattern of behavior (bar pressing and food ingestion have been most studied) or improved conflict resolution. Recent work documents the effect of ethanol on rhesus monkeys who are undergoing the stress of peer separations (Kraemer, Ebert, Lake, and McKinney, 1983; Kraemer, Lin, Moran, and McKinney, 1981). At low doses alcohol is effective in lessening the behavioral response to separation, whereas higher doses make the reaction more severe. Increasing attention to the utilization of paradigms that maximize the opportunities to study the potential beneficial, or harmful, role of alcohol on animals undergoing various kinds of stresses is indicated. It is an important clinical question and one that cannot easily, if at all, be investigated in humans.

Effect of Stress on the Intake of Ethanol

This complex area has been well summarized by Pohorecky. As mentioned earlier in this chapter, animals in general have a natural dislike for alcohol. The exceptions to this are certain alcohol-preferring strains of rats or mice that have been selectively bred for this purpose. A variety of procedures have been developed to increase ethanol intake by animals, and many of these have been previously reviewed in this chapter. They include such things as schedule-induced polydipsia, administration of diluted solutions as the source of fluid or as part of a liquid diet as the source of food, and stimulation of the lateral hypothalamus. Much has been learned from these studies regarding techniques to induce alcohol consumption in animals.

Physical stressors, in general, are ineffective. The most consistent results with behavioral stressors have been obtained when signaled unavoidable shock has been used with avoidance procedures. The results of a series of studies have been summarized by Pohorecky as follows:

> . . . many variables, including density of housing, sex of the animals, concentration of the solution of ethanol offered to the animals, duration of the experimental period, to name a few, make the evaluation and comparison of studies reviewed here difficult. Avoidance conditioning may elevate ethanol intake; however, the effects are moderate and rather short lived. In general, the most consistent results have been obtained when signaled unavoidable shock has been used with avoidance procedures. Clearly, if stressors play a role in overindulgence to ethanol in humans, the experimental approaches that have been attempted in animal research do not appear to be appropriate. Alternatively, rodents are not the appropriate animal species for this line of research. (1981, p. 220)

An illustration of recent research that attempts to deal with some of these issues used rhesus monkeys undergoing peer separations and found that the monkeys with the most severe behavioral response to separation increased their alcohol consumption the most and had the lowest baseline cerebrospinal fluid norepinephrine (Kraemer *et al.*, 1983). It is striking that two of the most powerful stressors, in terms of inducing increased alcohol intake in animals, are uncontrollability and separation paradigms, two of the paradigms being used to study some specific aspects of depressions.

Another interesting example which focuses on these interactions is a study by Pohorecky *et al.* (1981) of plasma levels of nonesterified fatty acids and corticosterone in rats. Stress alone markedly elevated these. Ethanol treatment alone also resulted in small elevations. However, when ethanol was given to stressed rats (the stress was footshock) the elevation of these substances was blocked. Thus, ethanol can affect stress-induced biochemical changes in experimental animals.

Drugs and Ethanol Intake

This area has been reviewed by Meisch (1977, 1982), who comments on the multiple methodological problems that prohibit general conclusions at this point. The most frequent strategy has been to administer ethanol by intubation, intraventricularly, or intravenously and to measure the effects of this exogenously administered ethanol on spontaneous alcohol consumption. In general, when ethanol is administered intravenously or by the intraperitoneal route, ethanol drinking is decreased. When alcohol is administered intraventricularly, the results have been mixed. Some studies have reported an increase in alcohol consumption, while others have reported no change.

The other strategy is to administer drugs which block the metabolism of acetaldehyde. These drugs, when administered systemically, decrease ethanol intake by rats and mice but have no effect on water intake. Chronic infusion into the ventricles of acetaldehyde, paraldehyde, methanol, and 5-hydroxytryptophol leads to increased ethanol drinking.

The effects of drugs which alter neurotransmitter system functioning on ethanol intake has been only minimally studied, and the results are mixed. (Cicero and Hill, 1970; Frey, Magnussen, and Nielsen, 1970; Geller, 1973; Geller, Purdy, and Merritt, 1973; Hill, 1974; Hill and Goldstein, 1974; Myers and Martin, 1973; Myers and Tytell, 1972; Myers and Veale, 1968; Myers, Evans, and Yaksh, 1972; Opitz, 1972; Veale and Myers, 1970). Clearly much more needs to be done in this area, since the complex interrelationships among neurotransmitter system function, reactions to stressors, and alcohol intake can be usefully investigated in animal paradigms.

As mentioned before, rats will generally increase their alcohol intake when exposed to psychological stress. In one study the stress was intermittent, random, unavoidable shock, and after exposure to this, rats significantly increased their alcohol intake. In this same study, the rats did not increase their alcohol intake when exposed to physiological stress. The elevation in alcohol preference was significantly reduced when PCPA was given but was unchanged when AMPT was given. Furthermore, the PCPA had a much greater effect on the animals designated as "high drinkers" than on those designated as "low drinkers." This effect of PCPA in psychologically stressed animals was different from its effects in nonstressed animals, where it lowered alcohol intake in rats which drank alcohol within the normal range of preference (Myers and Cicero, 1969).

Though PCPA is generally thought to decrease ethanol intake in rats, there is one study reporting no effect (Hill and Goldstein, 1974) and one reporting increased drinking (Geller, 1973). 5-hydroxytryptophan, a serotonin precurser, decreases ethanol drinking in rats (Geller, 1973; Geller *et al.*, 1973; Myers *et al.*, 1972). Intraventricular serotonin lowers ethanol, but not water, intake.

Over a range of doses, chlordiazepoxide results in increased drinking of both ethanol and water (Barrett and Weinberg, 1975). Trihexyphenidyl decreases ethanol drinking (Keehn, 1972).

Other Variables Influencing Ethanol Intake in Animals (Meisch, 1977, 1982)

1. *Sex differences*

   This has been the subject of many studies and reviews, and the details are beyond the scope of this chapter. In general, female rats drink more ethanol than male rats, and ethanol drinking increases during the estrus cycle. There is also a higher rate of ethanol metabolism in female rats.

2. *Order of Presentation and Schedule of Ethanol Access*

   An ascending series of concentrations leads to more ethanol consumption than a descending series and, in general, intermittent, as opposed to continuous, ethanol availability results in more ethanol drinking.

3. *Positive Reinforcement of Concurrent Behavior*

   This basically involves schedule-induced ethanol drinking. It has been obtained with mice, squirrel monkeys, rhesus monkeys, and rats. It has been possible to induce intoxication in this way, and the major technique used has been schedule-induced polydipsia. This has been previously discussed.

4. *Negative Reinforcement of Concurrent Behavior*

   This mostly involves lever pressing to avoid shock, and the data regarding possible increased alcohol consumption are inconsistent. In general, with rats, ethanol drinking is not significantly increased under conditions of negative reinforcement of concurrent behavior vs when concurrent behavior is positively reinforced and ethanol consumption goes up.

5. *Punishment of Concurrent Behavior*

   It is controversial whether noncontingent shock presentation in the absence of specifically reinforced concurrent behavior increases ethanol drinking or not.

6. *Food Deprivation*

Some aspects of this have been discussed previously. In general, ethanol intake of rats is increased by food deprivation. Reintroduction of free access to food leads to a decrease in ethanol intake to control levels or below. However, ethanol consumption systematically rises over a subsequent 20-day period until it exceeds control levels. Increasing the period of deprivation increases the ethanol drinking. Meisch states "the persistence of intake of high ethanol concentrations under conditions of food satiation suggests that ethanol drinking under conditions of food deprivation is not solely a function of ethanol's calories" (Meisch, 1977).

7. *Role of Physiological Dependence*

The establishment of physiological dependence is often given as one of the necessary criteria for demonstrating the validity of a given model of alcoholism. I disagree with this in that perfectly useful paradigms can be developed that may not involve physiological dependence at all yet may yield very useful information about the human alcohol problem. There are many clinically important questions about alcoholism that do not involve physiological dependence.

Even though physiological dependence can be demonstrated by a variety of methods in mice, rats, rhesus monkeys, and chimpanzees, the results consistently show that physiological dependence is not a necessary or sufficient condition for maintaining ethanol consumption. Ethanol can clearly serve as a reinforcer for rats that are not physiologically dependent.

8. *Miscellaneous Conditions Influencing Ethanol Intake in Animals*

Such things as the composition of the solution, the nature of the other liquids available, lighting, housing conditions, and temperature have all been studied in terms of how they influence ethanol intake and need to be considered in the design and analysis of a given experiment.

9. *Response Consequences*

Response consequences refers to the events that occur following emission of a specific response, usually operant in nature. These events have been less often considered in relation to studies of alcohol in animals, but the recent work of Meisch has highlighted their importance.

One concerns the schedules of reinforcement. Ethanol rein-

forcement (8%) will maintain fixed ratio, fixed interval responding for food deprived rats. Also, 8% and 22% ethanol will maintain FR responding of food satiated rats. The above pattern of
responding is similar to that maintained by more widely studied
reinforcers. 8% ethanol will also maintain FR responding of food
deprived rhesus monkeys.

Another response consequence concerns ethanol amount
used as a reinforcer. This can be varied by using a range of
concentrations and a constant volume per reinforcement or by
holding the concentration constant and varying the volume. In
rats and in rhesus monkeys, as the volume per reinforcement
increases, the number of reinforcements decreases. The same
finding holds with regard to volume.

Ethanol concentration has been mentioned in a number of
places in this chapter as an important variable, and many studies
are currently attempting to determine the effect of ethanol concentration on ethanol intake, time course of intake, and quantity
consumed. In general, rats will drink greater volumes of ethanol
than of water if the concentration is between 1.8% and 6%. They
will drink at concentrations above 6% if repeatedly presented an
ascending series of ethanol concentrations or if they are genetically selected for a predisposition to drink ethanol.

In conclusion to this section, it can be stated that alcohol is now
established as a reinforcer. Some of the variables involved in determining ethanol intake have now been studied. High ethanol intake can be
induced under conditions where less vehicle liquid is self-administered.
The opportunity to drink ethanol will maintain high levels of intermittently reinforced responding. Very few studies of a therapeutic sort have
been done which have attempted to eliminate ethanol drinking once it
has been established, nor have investigators begun to conceptualize
how to investigate the underlying mechanisms of the drinking patterns
of animals in these various paradigms. Cellular reductionism is not
needed as this area is approached, but rather a broad array of approaches is needed, including cellular ones, but also those involving
alternate methods to study mechanisms.

Alcohol Addiction in Monkeys and Young Chimpanzees

One of the themes pervading the animal–alcoholism literature is the
need for more primate studies and more focus on the behavioral stress-

inducing techniques. Developing these tools has not been easy, but some promising approaches have been developed, and many of these have been mentioned in the appropriate sections of this chapter.

Basically, monkeys have an aversion to alcohol and are not easily induced to consume it, although the work of Kraemer *et al.* with separated monkeys and aspartamate solutions indicates that this is not as true as was once thought (Kraemer *et al.*, 1983). Mello (1973), as well as other reviewers previously cited, has felt that efforts to develop behavioral methods to induce addictive drinking in rhesus monkeys have been unsuccessful for two reasons, namely, taste aversion and the delay between alcohol ingestion and intoxication, which "conceals" the potential reinforcing properties of oral alcohol ingestion. Monkeys will intravenously self-administer because of the immediacy of the effects obtained. For example, Mello and Mendelson reviewed some of their interesting experiments in which rhesus monkeys had to make a licking response to avoid shock (Mello and Mendelson, 1971). Both bourbon and ethanol solutions were presented in concentrations ranging from 5% to 25%. Each monkey would learn to drink to avoid shock at a rate sufficient to avoid virtually all possible shocks. However, the amount of fluid consumed decreased linearly as a function of increasing alcohol concentrations, even though the rate of responding remained the same. In other words, they learned to make a lick response to avoid the shock but modulated the amount of fluid drunk. The investigators then modified the apparatus so that only discrete licks of a specified duration were effective in postponing shock. The lick durations thus increased, but despite this, the volume of alcohol did not increase. They drank about 2.5 g/kg/day, and blood alcohol levels ranged between 30 and 70 mg/100 ml. No monkey showed evidence of intoxication or physical dependence.

By the use of polydipsia paradigms in monkeys, and using relatively low alcohol concentrations, more intoxication can be induced and larger volumes consumed. Thus, though the optimal parameters of schedule-induced ethanol consumption to produce self-intoxication are not yet clear, the data suggest a procedure involving multiple polydipsia sessions in which large volumes of low alcohol concentrations are consumed.

Another technique which is proving useful to produce increased alcohol intake in rhesus monkeys is peer separation. The quantities of alcohol self-selected by subgroups of monkeys undergoing this procedure is as high as recorded by any other measure, and whether eventual physiological dependence could be produced by this technique is not yet known (Kraemer *et al.*, 1983).

Alcohol addiction has been produced in young chimpanzees

(Pieper, Skeen, McClure, and Bourne, 1972). When they were 1–7 months old, they were given a liquid diet with 45% of the calories from ethanol, 4–5 times daily at standard feeding times. They maintained normal weight gain and consumed alcohol in doses from 2–8 g/kg. Blood alcohol levels ranged from 50–300 mg/100 ml, with peaks as high as 500 mg/100 ml depending on the concentration of alcohol in the liquid diet. They showed mild signs of withdrawal just prior to the morning feeding, after the 9-hour period since last feeding, when blood alcohol levels fell below 100–150 mg/100 ml. After 6–10 weeks of this regimen, the alcohol was abruptly withdrawn, and there were marked withdrawal symptoms. They also found an increased rate of ethanol metabolism as in humans, along with fatty infiltration of the liver.

This liquid diet procedure has been extended to adult rhesus monkeys with comparable results (Mello, 1973). They maintained 75–85% of ad lib weight and developed withdrawal signs after 155 days of consumption of 2.5–7 g/kg of alcohol presented in gradually increasing doses. Alcohol was administered twice daily, and withdrawal signs were frequently seen before the morning dose. Also, increases in the rate of ethanol metabolism were seen. In contrast to young chimpanzees, infant rhesus monkeys did not develop physical dependence after prolonged exposure to ethanol as the only fluid in an otherwise normal diet. This may be due to species differences or to a number of other factors. Obviously, if one wants to study physical dependence, this isn't the correct paradigm, although it may be enormously useful for other kinds of investigations relevant to alcoholism.

Summary of Key Points

- There is no such thing as an animal model of alcoholism, nor will there ever be.
- There has been significant progress in developing animal paradigms for the study of specific aspects of alcoholism.
- The use of forced administration techniques has made possible studies of alcohol metabolism, physical dependence, and withdrawal.
- The development of paradigms involving voluntary self-selection of alcohol permits the study of the motivational aspects of alcohol selection and the investigation of an important series of behavioral questions.
- These two fundamentally different approaches should not be criticized on the basis of not fulfilling certain criteria which themselves may be unre-

alistic. For example, even though most self-selection procedures do not lead to physical dependence, the continuing study of factors which influence alcohol consumption, even on an acute basis, is important. On the other hand, forced administration models should not be criticized on the basis that humans consume alcohol orally. That is true, of course, but the forced administration route may be the paradigm of choice in animals for studies of physical dependence and metabolism.

- *For the above, and other, reasons the term "animal model of alcoholism" should be dropped from our vocabulary, and the concept of suitable animal preparations for studying specific aspects of alcoholism should be substituted. The differences are more than semantic; they involve major concepts.*

- *The advantages and limitations of each type of preparation needs to be specified by the investigator, and this will be easier to do if there is no longer the attempt to be comprehensive.*

- *A type of animal preparation which needs to be developed and studied in more creative ways is one that will permit the study of the interaction between social stress factors and neurobiological factors in a variety of animals, especially primates. Little attention has been paid to this area, and the interaction of these variables is important in human alcoholism but impossible to study in a controlled way except in animal studies.*

- *Even if it is true that the initiation and course of alcohol intake in animals can never be made to parallel human alcohol intake exactly, the study of alcohol intake by animals can provide important insights into the relationships among the factors which control this behavior" (Amit, Sutherland, and White, 1975, p. 435).*

- *We should curb our nihilism and get on with the task at hand.*

References

Amit, Z., Stern, M. H. (1969) Alcohol Ingestion without Oropharyngeal Sensation. *Psychonomic Science* **15**:162–163.

Amit, Z., Amir, S., and Corcoran, M. E. (1973) A Possible Artifact in Studies of the Consumption of Ethanol by Rats. *Quarterly Journal of Studies on Alcohol* **34**:524–527.

Amit, Z., Sutherland, A., and White, N. (1975) The Role of Physical Dependence in Animal Models of Human Alcoholism. *Drugs and Alcohol Dependence* **1**:425–440.

Baker, T., and Cannon, D. (1982) Alcohol and Taste Mediated Learning. *Addictive Behaviors* **7**:211–230.

Barrett, J. E., and Weinberg, E. S. (1975) Effects of Chlordiazepoxide on Schedule-Induced

Water and Alcohol Consumption in the Squirrel Monkey. *Psychopharmacologia* **40**:419–328.

Cicero, T. J. (1980) Animal Models of Alcoholism. In *Animal Models in Alcohol Research*. K. Eriksson, J. D. Sinclair, and K. Anmaa (Eds.). London: Academic Press.

Cicero, T. J., Myers, R. D., and Black, W. C. (1968) Increase in Volitional Ethanol Consumption Following Interference with a Learned Avoidance Response. *Physiology and Behavior* **3**:657–660.

Cicero, T. J., and Hill, S. Y. (1970) Ethanol Self-Selection in Rats: A Distinction Between Absolute and 95% Ethanol. *Physiology and Behavior* **5**:787–791.

Clark, R., and Polish, E. (1960) Avoidance Conditioning and Alcohol Consumption in Rhesus Monkeys. *Science* **132**:223–224.

Conger, J. J. (1956) Reinforcement Theory and the Dynamics of Alcoholism. *Quarterly Journal of Studies on Alcohol* **17**:296–305.

Dember, W. N., and Kristofferson, A. B. (1955) The Relation Between Free-Choice Alcohol Consumption and Susceptibility to Audiogenic Seizures. *Quaterly Journal of Studies on Alcohol* **16**:86–95.

Deneau, G., Yanagita, T., and Seevers, M. H. (1969) Self-Administration of Psychoactive Substances by the Monkey. *Psychopharmacologia* **16**:30–48.

Deutsch, J. A., and Walton, N. Y. (1977) A Rat Alcoholism Model in a Free-Choice Situation. *Behavioral Biology* **19**:349–360.

Drewek, K. J., and Broadhurst, P. L. (1981) A Simplified Triple Testcross Analysis of Alcohol Preference in the Rat. *Behavior Genetics* **11(5)**:517–531.

Ellison, G. (1982) Novel Animal Model of Alcoholism Based upon Observation of Rats in Naturalistic Colony Environments (abstract). *Alcoholism: Clinical and Experimental Research*. D. H. Van Thiel (Ed.). **6**:294.

Ellison, G., Levy, A., and Lorant, N. (1983) Alcohol-Preferring Rats in Colonies Show Withdrawal, Inactivity, and Lowered Dominance. *Pharmacology, Biochemistry, and Behavior* **18**:565–570.

Eriksson, K. (1968) Genetic Selection for Voluntary Alcohol Consumption in the Albino Rat. *Science* **159**:739–741.

Eriksson, K. (1980) Inherited Metabolism and Behavior Towards Alcohol: Critical Evaluation of Human and Animal Research. In *Animal Models in Alcohol Research*, K. Eriksson, J. D. Sinclair, and K. Anmaa (Eds.). London: Academic Press.

Falk, J. L. (1961) Production of Polydipsia in Normal Rats by an Intermittent Food Schedule. *Science* **133**:195–196.

Falk, J. L. (1969) Conditions Producing Psychogenic Polydipsia in Animals. *Annals of the New York Academy of Sciences* **157**:569–593.

Falk, J. L. and Tang, M. (1980) Schedule Induction and Overindulgence. *Alcoholism: Clinical and Experimental Research* **4**:266–270.

Frey, H. H., Magnussen, M. P. and Nielsen, C. K. (1970) The Effect of p-Chloramphetamine on the Consumption of Ethanol by Rats. *Archives International de Pharmacodynamie et de Therapie* **183**:165–172.

Geller, I. (1973) Effects of Para-Chlorophenylalanine and 5-Hydroxytryptophan on Alcohol Intake in the Rat. *Pharmacology, Biochemistry, and Behavior* **1**:361–365.

Geller, I., Purdy, R., and Merritt, J. M. (1973) Alterations in Ethanol Preference in the Rat: The Role of Brain Biogenic Amines. *Annals of the New York Academy of Sciences* **215**:54–59.

Gorenstein, E. F., and Newman, J. P. (1980) Disinhibitory Psychopathology: A New Perspective and a Model for Research. *Psychological Review* **87**:301–315.

Greenberg, L., and Lester, D. (1953) The Effect of Alcohol on Audiogenic Seizures of Rats. *Q. Jl. Stud. Alcohol* **14**:385–390.

Hill, S. Y. (1974) Intraventricular Injection of 5-Hydroxytryptamine and Alcohol Consumption in Rats. *Biological Psychiatry* **8**:151–158.

Hill, S. Y., and Goldstein, R. (1974) Effect of *p*-Chlorophenylalanine and Stress on Alcohol Consumption by Rats. *Quarterly Journal of Studies on Alcohol* **35**:34–41.

Keehn, J. D. (1972) Effects of Trihexphenidyl on Schedule-Induced Alcohol Drinking by Rats. *Psychonomic Science* **29**:20–22.

Kraemer, G. W., Lin, D. H., Moran, E., and McKinney, W. T. (1981) Effects of Alcohol on the Despair Response to Peer Separation in Rhesus Monkeys. *Psychopharmacology* **73**:307–310.

Kraemer, G. W., Ebert, M. H., Lake, R., and McKinney, W. T. (1983) Neurobiological Measures in Rhesus Monkeys: Correlates of the Behavioral Response to Social Separation and Alcohol. In *Stress and Alcohol Use*, L. A. Pohorecky, and J. Brick, (Eds.). Amsterdam: Elsevier.

Lester, D., and Freed, E. X. (1973) Criteria for an Animal Model of Alcoholism. *Pharmacology, Biochemistry and Behavior* **1**:103–107.

Li, T. R., Lumening, L., McBride, W. J., and Waller, M. D. (1979) Progress toward a Voluntary Oral Consumption Model of Alcoholism. *Drug and Alcohol Dependence* **4**:45–60.

Masserman, J. H., and Yum, K. S. (1946) An Analysis of the Influence of Alcohol on Experimental Neuroses in Cats. *Psychosomatic Medicine* **VIII**:36–52.

Meisch, R. (1977) Ethanol Self-Administration: Infrahuman Studies. In *Advances in Behavioral Pharmacology*, T. Thompson and P. B. Dews (Eds.). New York: Academic Press.

Meisch, R. (1982) Animal Studies of Alcohol Intake. *British Journal of Psychiatry* **141**:113–120.

Meisch, R. A., and Thompson, T. (1971) Ethanol Intake in the Absence of Concurrent Food Reinforcement. *Psychopharmacologia* **22**:72–79.

Mello, N. K. (1973) A Review of Methods to Induce Alcohol Addiction in Animals. *Pharmacology, Biochemistry, and Behavior* **1**:89–101.

Mello, N. K. (1976) Animal Models for the Study of Alcohol Addiction. *Psychoneuroendocrinology* **1**:347–357.

Mello, N. K., and Mendelson, J. H. (1964) Operant Performance by Rats for Alcohol Reinforcement: A Comparison of Alcohol-Preferring and Nonpreferring Animals. *Quarterly Journal of Studies on Alcohol* **25**:226–234.

Mello, N. K., and Mendelson, J. H. (1966) Factors Affecting Alcohol Consumption in Primates. *Psychosomatic Medicine* **XXVIII**:529–550.

Mello, N. K., and Mendelson, J. H. (1971) The Effects of Drinking to Avoid Shock on Alcohol Intake in Primates. In *Biological Aspects of Alcohol*, M. K. Roach, W. McIsaac, and P. J. Creaven (Eds.). Austin: University of Texas Press.

Myers, R. D. (1966) Voluntary Alcohol Consumption in Animals: Peripheral and Intracerebral Factor. *Psychosomatic Medicine* **XXVIII**:484–497.

Myers, R. D. (1964) Modifications of Drinking Patterns by Chronic Intracranial Chemical Infusion. In *Thirst in the Regulation of Body Water*, M. J. Wayner (Ed.). Oxford: Pergamon.

Myers, R. D., and Carey, R. (1961) Preference Factors in Experimental Alcoholism. *Science* **134**:469–470.

Myers, R. D., and Cicero, T. J. (1969) Effects of Serotonin Depletion on the Volitional Alcohol Intake of Rats during a Condition of Psychological Stress. *Psychopharmacologia* **15**:373–381.

Myers, R. D., and Holman, R. B. (1966) A Procedure for Eliminating Position Habit in Preference-Aversion Tests for Ethanol and Other Fluids. *Psychonomic Science* 6:235–236.

Myers, R. D., and Martin, G. E. (1973) The Role of Cerebral Serotonin in the Ethanol Preference of Animals. *Annals of the New York Academy of Sciences* 215:135–144.

Myers, R. D., Stoltman, W. P., and Martin, G. E. (1972) Effects of Ethanol Dependence Induced Artificially in the Rhesus Monkey on the Subsequent Preference for Ethyl Alcohol. *Physiology and Behavior* 9:43–48.

Myers, R. D., and Tytell, M. (1972) Volitional Consumption of Flavored Ethanol Solution by Rats: The Effects of PCPA and the Absence of Tolerance. *Physiology and Behavior* 8:403–408.

Myers, R. D., and Veale, W. L. (1968) Alcohol Preference in the Rat: Reduction Following Depletion of Brain Serotonin. *Science* 160:1469–1471.

Myers, R. D., and Veale, W. L. (1972) The Determinants of Alcohol Preference in Animals. In *The Biology of Alcoholism Vol. 2: Physiology and Behavior*, B. Kissin, and H. Begleiter (Eds.). New York: Plenum.

Myers, R. D., Evans, J. E., and Yaksh (1972) Ethanol Preference in the Rat: Interactions Between Brain Serotonin and Ethanol, Acetaldehyde, Paraldehyde, 5-HTP, and 5-HTOL *Neuropharmacology* 11:539–549.

Newman, J. P., Gorenstein, E. E., and Kelsey, J. E. (1983) Failure to Delay Gratification Following Septal Lesions in Rats: Implications for an Animal Model of Disinhibitory Psychopathology. *Personality and Individual Differences* 4:147–156.

Opitz, K. (1972) Effects of Fenfluramine on Alcohol and Saccharin Consumption in the Rat. *South African Medical Journal* 46:742–744.

Orloff, E. R., and Masserman, J. H. (1975) Effect of Uncertainty on Emotionality and Ethanol Self-Selection in Monkeys with Cortical Ablations. *Biological Psychiatry* 10:245–251.

Orloff, E. R., and Masserman, J. H. (1978) Effects of Abstinence on Self-Selection of Ethanol Induced by Uncertainty in Monkeys. *Journal of Studies on Alcohol* 39:499–504.

Pieper, W. A., Skeen, M., McClure, H. M., and Bourne, P. G. (1972) The Chimpanzee as an Animal Model for Investigating Alcoholism. *Science* 176:71–73.

Pohorecky, L. A. (1981) The Interaction of Alcohol and Stress: A Review. *Neuroscience and Biobehavioral Reviews* 5:209–229.

Pohorecky, L. A., and Brick, J. (1977) Activity of Neurons in the Locus Coeruleus of the Rat: Inhibition by Ethanol. *Brain Research* 131:174–179.

Riley, E. P., Freed, E. X., and Lester, D. (1976) Selective Breeding of Rats for Differences in Reactivity to Alcohol. An Approach to An Animal Model of Alcoholism I. General Procedures. *Journal of Studies on Alcohol* 37:1535–1547.

Riley, E. P., Worsham, E. D., Lester, D. and Freed, E. X. (1977) Selective Breeding of Rats for Differences in Reactivity to Alcohol: An Approach to an Animal Model of Alcoholism II. Behavioral Measures. *Journal of Studies On Alcohol* 38:1705–1717.

Riley, A. L., Lotter, E. C., and Kulkosky, P. J. (1979) The Effects of Conditioned Taste Aversions on the Acquisitions and Maintenance of Schedule-Induced Polydipsia. *Animal Learning and Behavior* 7:3–12.

Rodgers, D. A. (1972) Factors Underlying Differences in Alcohol Preference of Inbred Strains of Mice. In *The Biology of Alcoholism*, B. Kissin and H. Begleiter (Eds.). New York: Plenum.

Rodgers, D. A., and McClearn, G. E. (1962) Mouse Strain Differences in Preference for Various Concentrations of Alcohol. *Quarterly Journal for Studies on Alcohol* 23:26–33.

Veale, W. L., and Myers, R. D. (1970) Decrease in Ethanol Intake in Rats Following Administration of p-Chlorophenylalanine. *Neuropharmacology* **9**:317–324.

Wallace, M. and Singer, G. (1976) Schedule-Induced Behavior: A Review of Its Generality, Determinants, and Pharmacological Data. *Pharmacology, Biochemistry, and Behavior* **5**:483–490.

Wayner, M. J., and Fisher, S. (1973) A Comparison of Ballpoint Drinking Sprouts and Richter Tubes in the Measurement of Ethanol Consumption. *Pharmacology, Biochemistry, and Behavior* **1**:351–352.

Wayner, M. J., and Greenberg, I. (1972) Effects of Hypothalamic Stimulation, Acclimation and Periodic Withdrawal on Ethanol Consumption. *Physiology and Behavior* **9**:737–740.

Wayner, M. J., Greenberg, I., Carey, R. J., and Nolley, D. (1971) Ethanol Drinking Elicited During Electrical Stimulation of the Lateral Hypothalamus. *Physiology and Behavior* **7**:793–795.

Wayner, M. J., Barone, F. C., and Jolicoeur, F. B. (1978) Effects of Ethyl Alcohol on Forced Consumption of an Acclimitated Saline Solution. *Pharmacology, Biochemistry, and Behavior* **8**:417–420.

Winger, G. D., and Woods, J. H. (1973) The Reinforcing Property of Ethanol in the Rhesus Monkey: I. Initiation, Maintenance, and Termination of Intravenous Ethanol-Reinforced Responding. *Annals of the New York Academy of Sciences* **215**:162–175.

Woods, J. H., Ikomi, F., and Winger, G. (1971) The Reinforcing Property of Ethanol. In *Biological Aspects of Alcohol*, M. K. Roach, W. McIsaac, and P. J. Creaven (Eds.). Austin: University of Texas Press.

Yanagita, T., and Takahashi, S. (1973) Dependence Liability of Several Sedative–Hypnotic Agents Evaluated in Monkeys. *Journal of Pharmacology and Experimental Therapeutics* **185**:307–316.

III

Perspectives on the Animal Modeling Field

III

Future Tasks

Introduction

In earlier sections of this book I have reviewed the history of the experimental psychopathology field and have also tried to provide a philosophical framework for its future development. These sections were followed by discussion of four representative clinical syndromes where attempts have been made to develop experimental animal models. These syndromes certainly do not represent a comprehensive examination of psychiatric syndromes where there is animal modeling research being conducted or where animal models could usefully be developed and potentially contribute to the progress of the field. They were chosen for reasons previously discussed, namely, because they illustrate many of the historical and philosphical points made in the first two sections of the book.

This section outlines what I see as some of the future directions the animal modeling field should take. It obviously represents my opinions alone, and others might see the situation quite differently. It is also likely to be the most controversial part of the book, although one can never be sure what of the other part might also strike tender nerves. However, this section in part deals with the interface between science and the politics of science in a way, to my knowledge, not done previously in this psychiatric research area.

I thought a long time before doing this, and considered having the book stay as strictly a scientific product dealing with the animal modeling of psychopathology research area with a focus on the interface with matters of clinical concern. Some, after reading this chapter, might wish that I had done so. However, the major threats to this research area are largely political and administrative rather than scientific. Despite a plethora of scientific advances in many areas of animal models of psychopathology (e.g., anxiety, depression, schizophrenia, substance abuse, dementias), the field remains scattered, fragmentary, and without a solid base of administrative or financial support. There are certainly things that workers in the field need to do to deal with the scientific issues. Many of these have been dealt with in previous chapters, but they are codified in this section. However, by and large, these tasks are being taken on, and progress in the area is as rapid, as in other areas of clinical psychiatric research, if not more so. Yet significant scientific and political problems remain. Why?

The Animal Rights Movement

All areas of biomedical research, from cancer to psychiatry, are under severe and extreme pressure from those who say they are concerned with animal rights. This is a rapidly growing movement in our country and abroad that opposes animal research, especially biobehavioral research. The movement is well organized and, seemingly, well-funded. Some moderates within this movement understand the value of animal research in medicine and want to insure that the care and treatment of animals in laboratories is humane. These goals are quite laudable and would be shared by animal researchers.

Unfortunately, the controversy has escalated from issues that can be rationally discussed and resolved in a mutually satisfactory manner to acts of physical violence. It is clear that the leadership of many of the organizations is antiscientific and extremist. Animal research laboratories have been broken into and animals released into situations where their survival would be problematic. There have been bombings and other terrorist tactics applied by those strongly opposed to the use of animals for any research purposes. Research laboratories have been infiltrated and misleading and selective photographic work done to try to document mistreatment of animals. It should be apparent that in this context any rational discussion of the issues is impossible.

What are the issues? One extreme view is that it is never defensible to use animals for biomedical research purposes. Those who hold this view would contend that any kind of cost-benefit analysis is useless. In this kind of analysis one basically asks the kinds of questions that are asked in research using human subjects, namely, do the potential benefits of the research outweigh the risks involved. It is not clear to me how those who hold this view expect medical research to proceed. I gather from their rhetoric that they do not expect it to continue or have some unrealistic expectation that computer simulations or other methodologies yet to be specified can replace the use of animals. They mention "alternatives" such as tissue cultures, radioimmunoassays, and computer modeling. It is interesting that these so called alternatives are, in actuality, research methods which have been developed by scientists as tools but which can never replace animal experimetation. For example, King (1984) has pointed out very effectively that radioimmunoassay techniques are really just new laboratory techniques just as any chemical analysis, but that "cell cultures, computers, and radioimmunoassays do not develop arthritis, blindness, diabetes, Alzheimer's disease, or any of the major health conditions which we need to study in their fully developed forms."

Unfortunately, this element of the animal rights movement seems to be very strong at present, very much influencing legislation, and attempting to intimidate researchers with threats of physical violence. Very little dialogue is possible in this kind of atmosphere. One of the future tasks, therefore, is to determine how best to deal with these elements. Certainly, we will have to stay vigilant and go on the offensive in terms of legislative initiatives to counter their efforts. If we do not, no amount of scientific advances will matter. A proud history of animal modeling research into major illnesses that includes development of the polio and other vaccines, development of anitdepressants and neuroleptics (drugs which have revolutionized the treatment of major psychiatric illnesses), techniques of doing renal transplants, cardiovascular surgical techniques, important immunological findings, development of insulin, and many other equally important health advances will be a thing of the past. This radical group has taken more time and has been far more effective than we have in making their case to the public and to legislators. We must work closely with organized medical and other professional groups to do a better political and public relations job.

There is no question that animal research has contributed greatly to advances in many fields of medicine, including psychiatry. Animal models are available for many illnesses and have been important in discoveries of important therapeutic advances. In addition to the examples given previously in this book, King (1984) has listed the following contributions within the field of behavior:

1. The use of biofeedback techniques in humans had their basic origins in the behavioral conditioning of so-called involuntary neuromuscular activities in rats and other animal species. Today,

biofeedback control of blood pressure is widely used to help prevent heart attacks and other sequelae of hypertension.

2. Language formation studies in the great apes has led to new concepts and practical methods in teaching language skills to severely retarded children and young people who, prior to this work, had no expressive language ability. As a result of animal research, many of these individuals can now express verbally for the first time their needs and feelings and can understand what others are saying to them.

3. Animal work on conditioned taste aversion has led to new and practical behavioral methods for helping those who have undergone radiation therapy for cancer to become interested in foods that are important for recovery.

4. Behavioral studies of the early development of vision in cats and primates, studies that could not have been done in children, have already led to new practices in pediatric ophthalmology that can prevent loss of vision in children with cataracts and strabismus.

5. Behavioral modification and behavioral therapy are now widely accepted techniques for modifying alcohol, drug, and tobacco addiction, obesity, and other health problems. They are a direct result of a long history of animal studies in learning theory and reward systems.

6. Programmed instruction, which is a valuable technique in educational and training programs, originated with operant learning studies in animals.

7. Results of primate studies in mother–infant bonding, depression, aggression, sexual development, infant abuse, and intellectual development have already begun to be incorporated into human child-rearing practices.

The above have represented major advances in the treatment of a variety of medical disorders and persist despite efforts of animal rights activists to downplay them. It is hard to believe that the public wants this kind of work to stop, yet that will be the result if present trends are not dramatically reversed.

It must be acknowledged that there have been some abuses of animals, just as there have been some abuses of human subjects in clinical research—yet no one is attempting to shut down clinical research. Of course, the abuses of animals should not have occurred, but they have been rare, given the history and the scope of animal modeling research. Reasonable improvements in the system of monitoring laboratory and field research with animals, some of which are already being implemented, should be supported by the scientific community. Instances of abuse, in addition to being unethical, do not help anyone and should be vigorously dealt with by peers and appropriate authorities.

The use of committees to review proposals involving the use of animals in research, much as human subjects committees review protocols involving human subjects, is indicated. Many institutions already have such review groups, and they are presently being developed as requirements at all places. This may seem like unnecessary administrative red tape to some, but, for both ethical and political reasons, it is indicated. Such groups need to look at the rationale for the research in terms of whether the procedures to which the animals are being subjected are justified by the research questions being asked. This is similar to a cost-benefit analysis done by human subjects committees. No research, human or animal, is not without potential risks or discomfort. The question is whether the risks are outweighed by the importance of the questions being asked. In addition, there needs to be attention paid to the degree of discomfort to which the animals (and humans in the case of human research) are to be subjected and how this is being handled in the protocol. The details of how such "animal subjects committees" should operate cannot be fully dealt with in this book, except to point out these developments, especially to clinicans, some of whom may be unaware of these changes in the animal modeling field.

Those researchers concerned with the development of animal models of psychopathology need to contemplate how to present their cases to such committees. Biomedical research relevant to psychiatric disorders has been especially controversial in some quarters of the animal rights movement and is poorly understood by others. This is one area where we need to be clear about what we are studying when we talk about, for example, an animal model of schizophrenia. Reference, in this regard, is made to the chapter on the philosophy of animal models and to the case examples discussed. We have a case to present which is as strong as that in any other field of medicine, and we should not hesitate to do so. A reasonable presentation might start with the importance of psychiatric disorders in terms of prevalence, morbidity, and mortality. Then, animal modeling research could be presented in the context of a variety of approaches to studying psychopathology. It could be pointed out how it complements clinical research in enabling us to study some factors that may be important but which cannot be studied in humans directly. Then, it can be mentioned that guidelines are now available, and others are being developed, which will help in careful application of the animal findings to our understanding of human psychopathology.

Some may need reminding that we are using animals to study selected aspects of human psychopathological syndromes, not modeling the entire syndrome. This approach is similar to that used in other fields of medicine. In my opinion, it is important to keep animal modeling of psychopathology research closely linked with other areas of biomedical research. At times in the past, it appears that this has not been so, and some in the animal rights movement would link psychopathological research more closely with "psychological research" and place it outside a medical context. In addition to being inaccurate, this is dangerous politically. We can use animal paradigms to study the etiology, pathogenesis, phenomenology, and treatment responsiveness of psychiatric illnesses with as much rationale and just as effectively as any other field of medicine.

Conceptual Tasks within the Field

Though many of our tasks are external and political, there are some issues within the field of animal modeling research that need to be addressed. Some of these, which were discussed previously in the chapter on the philosophy of animal models, are summarized here in addition to a few others. I hope that my colleagues who already understand all of this do not think that I am patronizing them. I certainly do not intend to. However, the field is diverse and includes people from many different disciplinary backgrounds. Also, many topics could be mentioned in such a section, and I cannot be comprehensive and keep this section to any manageable length. Therefore, the selection of tasks discussed may impress some as arbitrary, perhaps even random. There are many, but the following impress me as among the most important.

Development of a Basic Science of Animal Modeling

Since many disciplines are important to animal modeling in psychiatry, an interdisciplinary perspective is necessary. Animal modeling is far more complex than placing an animal in a certain situation, observing its behavior, and giving it a clinical label. There has been far too much of this in the history of the field already. The perspectives of a broad variety of fields needs to be brought to bear on the issue of animal modeling. Prominent among these, in addition to psychiatry, would be ethology, anthropology, experimental psychology, biostatistics, genetics, and the basic neurosciences.

What is needed is a set of guidelines, developed from an interdisciplinary perspective, about what animal models of psychopathology are, and are not, along with a framework to help guide future development of this still growing field. Such a perspective should include a framework about how to properly interpret experiments in animals in relation to their potential significance for human psychopathology. This is the perspective that has been largely missing from the animal modeling field and is very much needed in order to keep pace with rapid technological and methodological advances in experimentation.

Mainstreaming within Psychiatry

Animal modeling research relevant to psychopathology needs to be brought closer into the mainstream of contemporary psychiatry, as is medical and surgical research utilizing animals in their respective fields. This separation takes a number of forms as illustrated by the following examples.

Most of the leading mainstream psychiatric journals are very hesitant to publish articles using only animal subjects. Such articles are viewed as "basic science" and not particularly clinically relevant. Therefore animal modeling research ends up being published in basic science journals which are generally not read by most clinicians. The separation of clinical psychopathology research and animal modeling research is thus enhanced. One solution which has been considered is a new journal devoted to articles about animal modeling or comparative psychiatry. There are advantages and disadvantages to this type of solution. On the negative side is the fact that the market is already flooded with journals, and the last thing needed is a new journal. It is also not clear whether a journal would integrate clinical research about psychopathology with animal research on this same topic. On the plus side is the possibility of bringing together in one journal much of the animal modeling research about psychopathology. This work is presently scattered in basic psychology, psychopharmacological, behavioral, and other, journals. Such a journal could also provide a forum for continuing dialogue about some fundamental conceptual and philosophical issues in this emerging field of comparative psychiatry.

The separation is also illustrated in a different area, namely, the review and program administration of grants at the federal level. There are some conceptual issues that transcend the tight money issue. It is true that a number of animal models from many fields have been squeezed out in recent years, probably secondary to pressure from the animal rights movement, the expense involved in longitudinal maintenance of such preparations, and the increasing emphasis on molecular studies which as yet cannot be done in many animal preparations, especially in the psychiatric area. However, there is a special issue in the mental health area. Most institutes at NIH are comfortable with review groups composed of clinical–researchers and basic scientists reviewing both clinical research using humans and animal research about the appropriate illness. This is not so at NIMH, where there is a sharp separation at both the review and program administration levels between programs using humans as subjects and those with animals as subjects, pretty much independent of the content of a proposal. Animal research is viewed as "basic" and is assigned to basic science review committees. A more appropriate conceptualization would be for the assignment to be made based on the question being studied rather than the nature of the subjects being used. For example, a proposal using rodents as subjects but concerned with animal modeling of schizophrenia would be reviewed by a clinical psychopathology study section rather than a basic psychopharmacology section. I do not want in this book to spend too much time on the intricacies and politics of the grant review process or the territorial struggles involved in determining program administration issues. Such matters are more appropriate for other settings. The only reason for referring to them here is that they illustrate in a very real way the current separation between "clinical" research and "animal" research, a separation that is more typical of psychiatry than other specialties where there is more of a tradition of easier back and forth between the clinics and animal laboratories. The reasons for this separation have been discussed in earlier chapters and involve matters of history, tradition, and philosophy. It is hoped that as we move closer to the development of a solid base for a new area within psychiatry— comparative psychiatry—these barriers can become more permeable and less rigid.

As part of this rapprochement, workers in animal modeling research areas need to be thoughtful about how to improve linkages with the broader field of clinical psychiatry. From a historical standpoint, experimental techniques have been used which seem foreign to most clinicians, and clinical labels have been prematurely applied to animals' behaviors without careful enough attention having been paid to the context and meaning of the behaviors. We have often not spent enough time building the bridges necessary to establish better communication with clinicians necessary to establish better communication with clinicians about the value of animal research in psychiatry. This is clearly changing as evidenced by a number of recent developments, including an increasing recognition of past and present contributions of animal biobehavioral research to clinical psychiatry and the promises for the future. Many examples of such contributions have been mentioned, and more are given in the concluding chapter.

Recognition of the Interactive and Multivariate Nature of Psychopathology

This topic is extremely important for the next stage of our understanding of human psychopathology, and one in which animal modeling research can play a critical role.

Few would disagree in theory with the statement that most, if not all, forms of human psychopathology are determined by multiple variables. We do not have, and never will have, a single etiology for most psychiatric syndromes, or for that matter most illnesses in medicine in general. A series of variables can each have main effects accounting for some of the variance but also have interactions with each other to account for another proportion of the variance. This is a startlingly easy concept on first glance but one which most of us have trouble with in clinical practice and in research. There has been very little application of multivariate models or other analytic methods to our understanding of psychiatric illnesses. We are not yet able to be specific about how variables might interact to help produce a final result or even to obtain the empirical data that they do. Our statistical and conceptual models are sorely lacking in this area, yet a proper integration of an emerging body of genetic, developmental, social, personality, and neurobiological data awaits the development and/or application of such tools.

It has been difficult in human subjects to do research which focuses on the interactive effects of several variables. Conceptualizations about psychiatric illnesses, therefore, often are based on deterministic univariate reasoning. To talk about several variables interacting is often viewed as fuzzy thinking that is usually without, for methodological reasons, empirical support. Integrative models which involve multiple variables have been proposed for mood disorders (Whybrow, Akiskal, and McKinney, 1984) and for schizophrenia (Strauss and Carpenter, 1981), but most still find it difficult to truly operate either conceptually or clinically from these frameworks.

What does the field of animal modeling research have to contribute to this problem that is of relevance to clinicians? Quite simply, by developing appropriate experimental paradigms in animals, we can study prospectively the effects of a single variable or multiple variables. For example, when a variety of animals are subjected to situations in which they have no control over what happens to them (uncontrollability paradigms), they develop a series of behavioral disturbances. However, it has now been well established that the behavioral reactions in uncontrollability paradigms are heavily influenced by the neurobiological status of the animals at the time they are subjected to this particular inducing condition. The behavioral changes in response to being subjected to uncontrollability paradigms may or may not occur, depending on neurobiological variables. However, the neurobiological alterations alone may or may not lead to changes in behaviors, depending on what behavioral paradigms the animals are subjected to. Without having to draw parallels with any single clinical syndrome, this example illustrates how two kinds of variables, one neurobiological and the other situational, can interact to lead to altered behavior. Research utilizing animal paradigms has provided empirical data to support the importance of this interactive principle which may be important in many forms of human psychopathology.

Another example could be drawn from the clinical and animal literature on object loss or separation. This has been reviewed in more detail in an earlier chapter, but a part of this work is particularly relevant to this section on integrative and multivariate models of psychopathology and how animal research can help in this contest. It has been well documented from both human and animal research that attachment bond disruption at certain ages can have powerful and long-term behavioral effects. There are significant developmental influences on the responses to separation. More recent data from animals would support an interactive conceptualization of object loss much like it does the reaction to uncontrollability paradigms. To illustrate this point, there is individual variability in the reaction to separations in humans and in animals. The status of certain neurobiological systems at the time of separation influences the reactions to such losses and, conversely, the effects of certain drugs on both neurotransmitter systems and on behavior is significantly different, depending on whether they are given when the animals are together or when they are undergoing separations. Object loss or separations are complex events, and, again, we do not have to link this type of paradigm with any one form of psychopathology. It is one kind of paradigm for studying how a stressful event can influence neurobiological and behavioral functioning as well as responses to drugs, and, conversely, how the neurobiological status of an animal at the time it is subjected to a stressful situation can influence its behavioral reaction and account for some of the individual variability in response. Understanding such interactions is fundamental to developing improved treatment strategies and helping people deal with such stressors. It is only by such gradual advancement that we will make progress in developing a data-based, truly integrative view of some fundamental issues in psychopathology. Research utilizing animal models has a key role to play in this area.

One of the future tasks for researchers working in the animal modeling area is to develop some improved and creative paradigms for studying this interaction among the multiple variables involved in psychopathology. Many paradigms are available and could be further developed along these lines. New ones could be developed. To do this will require close and ongoing interaction with clinical researchers concerned with psychopathology in humans. This is another example of why it is critical to foster the interface between animal modeling research and clinical psychopathology research. We are not necessarily even talking about modeling a certain clinical syndrome in animals; rather, the interest is in developing some experimental paradigms to evaluate some fundamental principles in human psychopathology.

Recognition of the Limitations of Animal Modeling Research

Just as it is important to be clear about the actual and potential contributions of animal research in relation to psychopathology, it is equally important to be aware of its limitations. This has been an issue in the past, and it remains one of our future tasks. Those outside the field are not shy about pointing out the limitations of animal modeling or, on the other hand, having unrealistic expectations. Where is the proper middle ground?

As mentioned several times in this book, we must be extremely cautious about cross-species reasoning. Generalizations of results directly from one species to another are not justified without apropriate attention being paid to species differences as well as to differences in the context and meaning of the behaviors. However, there may be the suggestion of some fundamental principles relevant to another species, the further study of which may be indicated in that species. Examples of this have been given already.

One of the future tasks is to avoid the premature application of clinical labels to syndromes in animals despite their apparent behavioral similarity to those seen in humans with certain forms of psychopathology. This involves the increasing recognition that we are limited in terms of what we can model in animals. We can never model a human psychiatric illness totally. If this could be done it would no longer be a model. It would be the real thing. Perhaps this is not a limitation so much as a reconceptualization of what models are or are not. We might wonder if we should scrap the whole term "animal model" in recognition of this limitation, yet if it is recognized that animals can be used to study some specific issues relevant to human psychopathology without having to model the whole syndrome, the term can be kept. Additional specific limitations in this regard are discussed earlier in this book.

Special attention should be paid in this regard to both the advantages and limitations of animal models for doing mechanism studies. Our field is fond of coining terms, and the latest is "molecular psychiatry." Can you imagine terms such as "molecular pediatrics" or "molecular medicine"? While few would deny the importance of understanding behavior at all levels, some in our field specifically evaluate animal models by how suitable they are for conducting molecular mechanistic studies. What is meant by such a requirement is rarely clear, and we need to be extremely careful in thinking through what type of mechanism study is appropriate for which paradigm. For example, if we are studying invertebrates, fairly direct studies of neuronal functioning can be done. There are tremendous advantages to such approaches. The limitation of such paradigms relates to what the behaviors mean and, therefore, the significance of the changes in neuronal functioning On the other hand, another paradigm might involve very sophisticated assessment of social behavior in primates but not a direct assessment of neuronal functioning. There are advantages and disadvantages in every paradigm discussed in this book, and one of the future tasks is to be clear about the contributions and limitations of each approach. Contentious debates about which is the "best" model for a given clinical syndrome are nonsensical, and if the field is going to continue to develop, these debates must cease.

References

King, F. (1984) Human Benefits and Current Problems in Behavioral Research with Animals. Symposium on Animal Rights and Behavior Analysis. Annual meeting of the Association for Behavioral Analysis, May, 1984. Nashville, TN.

Straus, J. S., Carpenter, W. T. (1981) *Schizophrenia.* New York: Plenum.

Whybrow, P. C., Akiskal, H., McKinney, W. T. (1984) *Mood Disorders: Toward a New Psychobiology.* New York: Plenum.

8

Conclusions

This has been a book about an old quest but also a new field within psychiatry. The quest dates back to at least the time of Thorndike and then of Pavlov, who developed the novel notion that it was more important to study actual behavior than to engage in endless speculation about inner states. These scientists proceeded to develop experimental paradigms in animals in a laboratory setting and to perform studies of "experimental neurosis."

In a somewhat broader context, of course, the writings of Darwin concerning the evolutionary basis of human behavior provided a context for the considerable work on experimental psychopathology which has followed. Melvin Konner, in his excellent book *The Tangled Wing*, provides an instructive perspective on Darwin's contributions to our understanding of adaptation, a concept central to our understanding of psychopathology in the laboratory or in everday life. It would take us far afield from the purpose of this book to discuss the concept of adaptation and what it means to evolutionary biologists, sociobiologists, biological anthropologists, etc. But Konner's book is highly recommended reading for psychiatric clinicians interested in the subject of this book, namely, animal models of psychopathology.

The present book has proposed that what has more traditionally been thought of as animal modeling of psychopathology be put in a somewhat broader context, namely, that of a new comparative psychiatry. This newly conceptualized field would certainly include animal modeling work but would also recognize the exploding knowledge base in such basic sciences as ethology, sociobiology, anthropology, paleontology, and comparative psychology that is assuming considerable relevance for psychiatry. Developing the interface of psychiatry with such fields would put animal modeling work on a more solid footing than has sometimes been true historically, where manipulations have been made and the resultant behaviors given clinical labels. It would help us learn to reason across species. Konner has put it well when he points out that baboons or chimpanzees or any other higher primate species "can only constitute one set of data points in the panorama of higher primate behavior."

> Only after many data points have yielded an overall structure can we derive general principles, and only from such principles can we make any guesses about our ancestors. Baboons, chimpanzees, and people are what they are because of unique histories of evolutionary demands. Understanding will come not from a comparison of ourselves with another primate species but from establishment of the general laws that have brought about all our uniquenesses.*

Konner goes on to point out that cross-species reasoning in the realm of behavior is really no different from that applied to certain anatomical parts, in that one begins with comparative studies where there are known degrees of relatedness and then generalizes from principles that are derived from this comparison along with some elementary assumptions about the uniformity of the process of evolution.

Unfortunately, the history of the animal modeling field is filled with examples of writings that illustrate the failure to understand some basic principles of evolutionary theory and of animal behavior. This problem continues today in our search for molecular mechanisms without understanding the behaviors themselves.

Therefore, a key step in the future development of the comparative psychiatry field is an improved understanding of the basic sciences of animal modeling and their incorporation into the mainstream of psychiatry. This will have to unfold gradually, just as the basic sciences of clinical psychopharmacology have developed gradually and the interface expanded over time.

This relates to what has been another key point in the present book, namely, a clarification of the philosophical basis for the development of animal models for any psychiatric illness. This involves a definition of models and an understanding of the different types of models. In this book, animal models have been viewed as experimental preparations developed in one species for the purpose of studying phenomena occurring in another species. One does not develop an animal model for any syndrome. The more proper conceptualization is that of developing a number of specific preparations for studying aspects of psychopatho-

---

*Melvin Konner, *The Tangled Wing* (1982), New York: Harper & Row, p. 33.

logical syndromes. One can never model a syndrome in its entirety in animals.

A distinction has been made between models designed to simulate specific signs or symptoms of the disorder, those designed to evaluate specific etiological theories, those designed to study underlying mechanisms, and those designed primarily to permit preclinical drug evaluations. Though there may be overlap in some cases, the primary purpose for developing the model is different. Evaluation of models needs to relate to the purpose for developing them in the first place.

In Part II, four illustrative case examples have been given. These include affective disorders, schizophrenic disorders, anxiety disorders, and alcoholism. In the case of each syndrome, there have been a number of approaches to creating and utilizing animal models that are relevant to both clinicians and basic scientists.

There are many challenges that confront this newly emerging field of comparative psychiatry, one component of which is animal modeling. There are a significant number of basic sciences involved, and their literature is equally important to psychiatry as to the neurosciences. I think the future will see an increasing interest in this interface, and this book is one attempt to begin this process, with its focus on the area of animal modeling of psychopathology.

Index